Aging and Money

Ronan M. Factora
Editor

Aging and Money

Reducing Risk of Financial Exploitation and Protecting Financial Resources

Second Edition

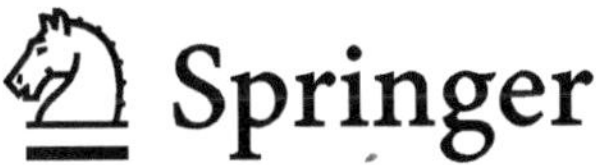

Editor
Ronan M. Factora
Cleveland Clinic Lerner College of Medicine at Case Western Reserve University
Cleveland Clinic, Cleveland, OH, USA

ISBN 978-3-030-67564-6 ISBN 978-3-030-67565-3 (eBook)
https://doi.org/10.1007/978-3-030-67565-3

This Springer imprint is published by the registered company Springer Nature Switzerland AG
The registered company address is: Gewerbestrasse 11, 6330 Cham, Switzerland

Preface

This book came about after a collaboration between me and my geriatric medicine colleagues after presenting a symposium on financial exploitation at the American Geriatrics Society Scientific Meeting in 2012. The interest that came out following this symposium demonstrated how concerned my colleagues were about this issue, and discussions with professionals from other disciplines showed they had similar concerns.

Increasingly, older persons have been targeted as potential victims to be taken advantage of for their financial resources. Individuals from the lowest income brackets to multimillionaires, from the next-door neighbors to famous faces, have become victims of financial exploitation. Though this form of elder abuse has been recognized for years, its incidence, prevalence, and impact on the common individual continues to be a challenge to identify and address. In the context of the great recession and the baby-boomer population reaching retirement age, the temptation to take advantage of these elders who are trusting, disabled, or cognitively impaired may be greater now than at any other time. We now know that the increased risk in this population has a physiological underpinning as we continue to understand more about how structural and functional changes in the brain are associated with higher risk of victimization.

Despite all of the advancing knowledge, recognition of risk factors and indicators of financial exploitation are not widely disseminated. Additionally, once financial exploitation is identified and confronted, the knowledge of what to do next is also lacking. Many resources are available, but lack of awareness of their existence is a significant barrier to their use. These gaps are present within the medical community, law-enforcement, and the financial community – areas where opportunities for recognition and intervention are common. Our elders often have no idea of what to do when they see their own risk or when they fall victim.

The purpose of this book is to help disseminate and share knowledge about this problem with the purpose of protecting those individuals in our society who are vulnerable to financial abuse and exploitation. This edition seeks to highlight the perspectives of those who encounter this problem in different disciplines, including professionals in medicine, law, the financial industry, and social services.

Understanding what each discipline's role is in investigating and managing this issue is a key to achieving success. With this knowledge, the reader can look to their own community to seek out local champions to fight for the cause and join those across the nation who work for the same goal.

Cleveland, OH, USA Ronan M. Factora

Acknowledgments

I would like to thank the many collaborators whose names grace the pages of this work. They represent a small number of a dedicated cadre of professionals whose focus is the protection of the frailest and most vulnerable, the most venerable of our community.

Contents

Contributors

Lori Albee, MVSM The Texas Department of Family and Protective Services, Adult Protective Services, Houston, TX, USA

Georgia J. Anetzberger, PhD, ACSW, FGSA Schools of Applied Social Sciences and Medicine, Case Western Reserve University, Cleveland, OH, USA

Jason Beaman, DO, MS, MPH, FAPA Department of Psychiatry and Behavioral Sciences, Oklahoma State University Center for Health Sciences, Tulsa, OK, USA

Lisa J. Bleier SIFMA, Washington, DC, USA

Celiza P. Bragança Bragança Law LLC, Skokie, IL, USA

Jason Burnett, PhD Internal Medicine, Division of Geriatric and Palliative Medicine, The University of Texas Health Science Center at Houston, (UTHealth), McGovern Medical School, Houston, TX, USA

Anthony Casacchia, MD Division of Geriatric Medicine, Summa Health System, Akron, OH, USA

Jennifer Drost, DO, MPH Division of Geriatric Medicine, Summa Health System, Akron, OH, USA

Natalie C. Ebner Department of Psychology, University of Florida, Gainesville, FL, USA

Institute on Aging, Department of Aging & Geriatric Research, University of Florida, Gainesville, FL, USA

Cognitive Aging and Memory Clinical Translational Research Program, University of Florida, Gainesville, FL, USA

Florida Institute for Cybersecurity Research, McKnight Brain Institute, & Pain Research and Intervention Center of Excellence, University of Florida, Gainesville, FL, USA

Ronan M. Factora, MD Cleveland Clinic Lerner College of Medicine at Case Western Reserve University, Cleveland Clinic, Cleveland, OH, USA

Renee J. Flores, MD Internal Medicine, Division of Geriatric and Palliative Medicine, The University of Texas Health Science Center at Houston, (UTHealth), McGovern Medical School, Houston, TX, USA

Adam M. Fried, Esq. Reminger Co. LPA, Cleveland, OH, USA

Probate and Trust Litigation, Cleveland, OH, USA

Gerson Galdamez, PhD Leonard Davis School of Gerontology, University of Southern California, Los Angeles, CA, USA

Diana Homeier, MD University of Southern California, Los Angeles, CA, USA

Natalie Kayani, MD Division of Geriatric Medicine, Summa Health System, Akron, OH, USA

Bonnie E. Levin Alexandria and Bernard Schoninger Professor of Neurology, University of Miami, Miller School of Medicine, Miami, FL, USA

Franklin C. Malemud, Esq. Reminger Co. LPA, Cleveland, OH, USA

Probate and Trust Litigation, Cleveland, OH, USA

Carol A. Miller, MSN, BC Care and Counseling, Brecksville, OH, USA

Aanand D. Naik Professor and Chief, Section of Geriatrics and Palliative Medicine, Department of Medicine, Baylor College of Medicine, Houston, TX, USA

Gretchen Napier Life-Links Geriatric Care Management, Nashville, TN, USA

Sharlene Nauls, LMSW The Texas Department of Family and Protective Services, Adult Protective Services, Houston, TX, USA

James S. Powers, MD Center for Quality Aging, Vanderbilt University School of Medicine, Nashville, TN, USA

Tennessee Valley Geriatric Research, Education, and Clinical Center, Nashville, TN, USA

Robert E. Roush, EdD, MPH Baylor College of Medicine, Houston, TX, USA

Julia Margaret Rowan, PhD Leonard Davis School of Gerontology, University of Southern California, Los Angeles, CA, USA

Carolyn K. Smith, LCSW Tennessee Valley Healthcare System, Nashville, TN, USA

Sherif Soliman, MD Forensic and Geriatric Psychiatry, Atrium Health, Charlotte, NC, USA

R. Nathan Spreng Laboratory of Brain and Cognition, Montreal Neurological Institute, Department of Neurology and Neurosurgery, McGill University, Montreal, QC, Canada

Departments of Psychiatry and Psychology, McGill University, Montreal, QC, Canada

Douglas Mental Health University Institute, Verdun, QC, Canada

McConnell Brain Imaging Centre, McGill University, Montreal, QC, Canada

Timothy L. Takacs, JD, CELA Takacs McGinnis Elder Care Law, PLLC, Hendersonville, TN, USA

Gary R. Turner Department of Psychology, York University, Toronto, ON, Canada

Page B. Ulrey King County Prosecutor's Office, Seattle, WA, USA

Chapter 1
Facts and Figures

Ronan M. Factora

Overview

> With good reason, financial elder abuse has been characterized by some experts as "the crime of the 21st Century [1].

Exploitation and abuse of older persons is a phenomenon that spans centuries, continents, and cultures. The United States started to publically recognize and legislatively address financial exploitation of this group of people in the latter half of this century, long after work on child abuse and violence against women was advocated and underway. With the "graying of America," there has never been such a crucial time to develop a full understanding of this phenomenon and to continue to develop appropriate interventions to prevent exploitation and injury to this often vulnerable segment of our society. This chapter will review the demographics of financial exploitation in this population, the impact on the victims of such abuse, and the legislative response to this growing phenomenon.

Aging in the United States and Risk of Financial Exploitation

Americans are living longer and in increasing numbers with the aging of the baby boomer generation. There were 52 million people over 65 years of age according to a 2018 census, and by the year 2050, this number will exceed 80 million, of which 19% will be over the age of 85. Consequently, there will be a rise in the numbers of individuals living in a frail, dependent, and debilitated state, with associated

R. M. Factora (✉)
Cleveland Clinic Lerner College of Medicine at Case Western Reserve University, Cleveland Clinic, Cleveland, OH, USA
e-mail: factorr@ccf.org

R. M. Factora (ed.), *Aging and Money*,
https://doi.org/10.1007/978-3-030-67565-3_1

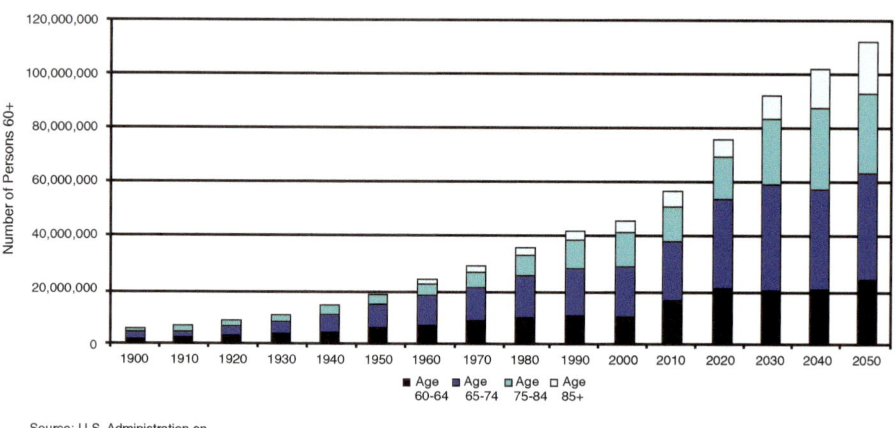

Fig. 1.1 Increase in US population by age/year from 1900 to 2050. (Adapted from the US Administration on Aging using the census data from the Bureau of the Census)

increased monetary and societal costs. The National Aging Information Center projected that the number of individuals with severe disability requiring partial or total assistance will increase from 3.8 million in 1990 to 14.3 million by the year 2040, with 70% expected to be over the age of 85 [2] (Fig. 1.1).

In the United States, most community-residing individuals with disabilities are cared for by families or paid caregivers. Currently, 5% of the elderly in the United States are in long-term care settings, with the majority being women and 22% over the age of 85. It is estimated that for every individual living in a nursing home, five individuals are cared for at home by family or paid caregivers. These changing demographics raise concern about a rising financial and social burden placed on a proportionately smaller younger generation of caretakers. It also represents a growing pool of potential elder abuse victims [3].

Definitions of Elder Abuse and Financial Exploitation

Elder abuse is a societal problem with domains cutting across social, clinical, criminal, business, and legal arenas. Although the disciplines of medicine and law define and detail abuse through their respective interests, expertise, and skills, broader working definitions have evolved to better define, label, and study the problems outside these specific professional venues to reach a larger audience and address the broader implications of social justice. The Center for Disease Control (CDC) defines elder maltreatment as "any abuse and neglect of persons age 60 and older by a caregiver or another person in a relationship involving an expectation of trust." [4] Further, the National Center on Elder Abuse (NCEA) defines seven types of elder maltreatment based on its analysis of existing state and federal definitions of elder abuse, neglect, and exploitation. The seven types of abuse defined by NCEA are as follows: physical abuse, sexual abuse, emotional abuse, financial/material exploitation, neglect, abandonment, and self-neglect. Detailed definitions are published on the NCEA's website. The NCEA's general definition of financial and material exploitation is the "illegal or improper use of an elder's funds, property, or assets" [5].

In the realm of the US federal law, the Older Americans Act of 2006 defined financial exploitation as "fraudulent or otherwise illegal, unauthorized, or improper act or process of an individual, including a caregiver of fiduciary, that uses the resources of an older individual for monetary or personal benefits, profit, or gain, or that results in depriving an older individual of rightful access to, or use of, benefits, resources, belongings, or assets" [6]. This federal statute speaks to a spectrum of financial exploitation in the United States. The exploitation the statute implies can range from blatantly criminal activity with explicit intent to defraud the victim to careless or unwise financial transactions by individuals or caregivers of the victim presented as necessary or normal behavior. What constitutes "improper" use of finances given the differences in cultural beliefs and mores further complicates the operationalization of the financial exploitation definitions, as perpetrators fall into several categories, ranging from trusted family and friends to financial advisors and total strangers.

Landmark US Studies of Elder Abuse Prevalence and Incidence

Measuring the scope of elder abuse, neglect, and mistreatment has been a monumental task. Early difficulties stemmed from lack of standardized definitions, absence of mandates for reporting such abuse or a central repository for such information, need for coordination and communication between agencies involved in this work, and standardized methodologies for advancing study and education in this area. The bulk of data derived from local surveys and community studies was extrapolated to national estimates. Over the past two decades, new methods of sampling and identifying elderly mistreatment have helped improve validity and comprehensiveness of elder mistreatment occurrence estimates. Several landmark studies have expanded our knowledge about elder abuse and have stimulated recent social and federal legislative changes.

The 1998 National Elder Abuse Incidence Study (NEAIS) was one of the first landmark studies exposing the scope of the problem of elder abuse and neglect in the United States. It published the first national estimates of its incidence. This study, funded as part of the 1992 Family Violence Prevention and Service Act and conducted with the National Center for Elder Abuse, collected data from state Adult Protective Services (APS) reports and investigations, as well as from "sentinels" in 248 community agencies [7]. Drawing on past study experience in child abuse studies, the NEAIS used "sentinels" to gather incidence data, as officially reported cases of abuse were felt to underreport the number of actual cases of elderly abuse and neglect. The sentinels in the NEAIS were specialty trained individuals who had regular contact with the elderly in multiple community agencies including law enforcement, hospitals and public health institutions, and elder care providers.

The NEAIS collected data in 20 counties in 15 states and reported that approximately 450,000 elderly persons aged 60 and above were abused or neglected in domestic settings during 1996. This incidence rate was up to five times higher than the incidence rate of reports to APS the same year. This suggested that up to 379,000 cases of elder abuse went unreported, with 35% of the cases of elderly abuse representing emotional abuse, financial exploitation (30%), physical abuse (26%), and abandonment (4%) (Fig. 1.2). The study showed that female elders experienced higher rates of abuse or neglect than males. The oldest old (> 80 years) were abused at 2–3 times the rate of the young old. In almost 90% of the abuse and neglect incidents, the perpetrator was a family member, with two-thirds of these being adult children or their spouses. Eighty-five percent of the perpetrators of financial exploitation were under 60 years of age.

The NEAIS provided a detailed risk profile of the victims and the kinds of abuse suffered. The profiles showed that 50% were unable to care for themselves, 60% had some form of cognitive decline, and 44% developed depression. Males were the

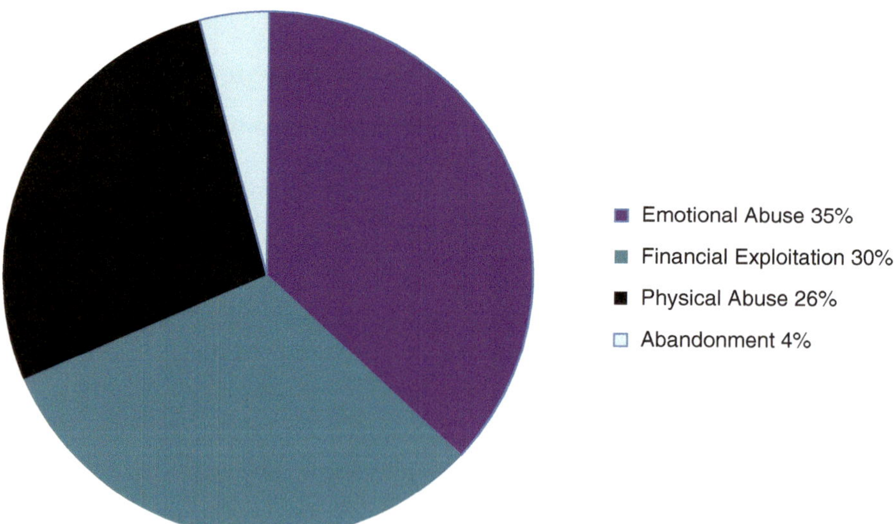

Fig. 1.2 Types of elder mistreatment. (Adapted from the National Elder Abuse Incidence study: Prepared for the Administration for Children and Families and the Administration on Aging in the US Department of Health and Human Services [7])

most frequent perpetrators for abandonment (84%), physical abuse (62%), emotional abuse (61%), and financial exploitation (59%). Females were more commonly involved in neglect (52%). White elders were the predominant victims for maltreatment, while black elders were more likely to be neglected or suffer from financial exploitation or emotional/psychological abuse.

Supporting the findings of the NEAIS study, the National Association of Adult Protective Services Administrators (NAAPSA) conducted a study of financial exploitation of vulnerable elders in 2001. They surveyed 34 states with 28 states reporting 15% of the substantiated reports involved financial exploitation at a prevalence of 38,015 within the last year. More than half of the victims were female, and the majority (64%) were 66 or older. A few states reported that the victims had higher incomes, but the majority found the victims had incomes similar to other APS clients. These same individuals, however, had greater real estate assets (property and non-monetary resources), which the perpetrators were more likely to target [8].

A further study in 2004 revealed an even higher estimate of victims, ranging from 100,000 to as high as one million per year, with reported cases up almost 20% from the first survey. Financial exploitation was the third most commonly substantiated form of elder abuse following neglect and emotional or psychological abuse. Again, females emerged as the most common victims, with 42.8% over the age of 80. The majority were Caucasians. Perpetrators were more likely to be adult children or other family members, female, and younger (age less than 60) [9]. Additionally, Laumann et al. appended the National Social Life, Health, and Aging project with questions of mistreatment [10]. The study surveyed 2005 elderly, thought to be nationally representative sample. It found a past year prevalence of verbal abuse (9%), financial mistreatment (3.5%), and physical abuse (0.2%). The demographics were similar to prior studies, with women and physically frail individuals far more likely to suffer verbal mistreatment. African Americans were more likely to report financial exploitation. The cumulative conclusions of these more recent studies show a clear increase in elder mistreatment of all forms, with an emerging trend toward financial exploitation. The pattern for victims remained consistent, with women and the old-old being the targets for abuse and perpetrators most likely family members, typically adult children.

Consumer fraud has increasingly become common. A report from the Federal Trade Commission provided to Congress in October 2019 [11] provided the following key findings:

- Though older individuals were less likely to be targets of fraud, when it does occur in an older person, the dollar amount of loss is higher compared to younger adults.
- Losses increased based on the age of the individual.
- Phone scams were the most "lucrative" against older consumers.
- Older individuals were more likely compared to younger individuals to report victimization through tech support scams, prize, sweepstakes & lottery scams, and family & friend impersonation.

The Many Faces of Financial Exploitation – A Profile of the Victims

"My money was stolen from me, by someone close," entertainment legend Mickey Rooney, 90, testified in front of a Senate Special Committee on Aging hearing exploring the nationwide trends of abuse, neglect, and financial exploitation. Rooney filed a restraining order against his stepson and stepdaughter, claiming both emotional and financial abuse, and alleging he was locked up in his house and given no explanation why his rights were stripped of him.

The disgraced son of Brooke Astor, a prominent New York socialite, Anthony Marshall was convicted in 2009 of grand larceny for taking advantage of his mother with dementia and plundering her $200 million fortune. Anthony Marshall's son filed a lawsuit against him claiming that his father had not provided for his elderly mother who suffered from Alzheimer's disease. Instead, he allowed her to live in squalor and failed to provide necessary medication and doctor's visits while enriching himself with income from her estate. The grandson requested a change in guardianship to Annette de la Renta, the wife of designer Oscar de la Renta.

These high-profile cases bring much renewed national and international publicity to the issues of financial exploitation of the elderly. However, as reported in the MetLife news feeds, this form of elder abuse spans across all classes, races, and cultures and frequently occurs in obscurity and therefore draws little attention. Even more so than other forms of abuse, precise measurement of financial exploitation of the elderly across cultures is difficult to determine, as varied cultures have vastly differing attitudes and norms regarding what constitutes improper use of funds.

In the United States, people in their late 70s and 80s were shaped by their experiences during the great depression. They currently represent the wealthiest cohort of Americans, with their wealth estimated to be $1–3 trillion or 70% of the nation's assets [12]. Physical dependency and cognitive decline are the predominant attributes that make older persons vulnerable to abuse and exploitation. These physical and cognitive vulnerabilities coupled with this cohort's trusting character and unprecedented financial wealth have created a prime target for financial exploitation.

The "typical victim" of financial exploitation in the United States is described by APS as an elderly female, Caucasian, between the ages of 70 and 89, physically frail, and/or cognitively impaired [7]. Other studies confirm that women over the age of 70 are at highest risk for exploitation [13–15]. Additionally, living with a caregiver or being socially isolated or widowed increases one's vulnerability to financial exploitation [9, 12, 15].

Racial differences in financial exploitation in the United States found that African Americans have a significantly higher rate of financial exploitation than Caucasians and Latinos, but Latino's were less likely to report any type mistreatment [10]. In fact, African Americans had nearly four times greater risk for financial exploitation than non-African Americans and an 8.5-fold risk of occurrence within the last 6 months of life. The majority of these perpetrators were not family members [16].

Cognitive decline represents a major risk factor for financial exploitation and can occur before frank dementia is diagnosed. This vulnerability occurs not only because of poor financial judgment but also because of diminished ability to detect or prevent exploitation. With progressive cognitive loss, there is an increased dependency on others for assistance in financial management, exposing these individuals to potentially greater risk of financial exploitation. Recent research on the neurobiology of aging shows that even early cognitive changes can increase the risk of financial exploitation. A study found that persons with mild cognitive impairment (MCI) were four times more likely to make financial errors than those without MCI [17]. Damage from strokes or degenerative process to the orbitofrontal cortex (OFC), the part of the brain that houses executive function and judgment, can result in less risk-aversive behavior. Additionally, a sizable portion of older adults (approximately 45%) perform poorly on measures of financial decision-making with marked changes in responses to risk taking, ambiguity, and reaction to rewards or punishment and may have more likelihood to fall prey to exploitation [18].

In addition to individual vulnerabilities, interpersonal dynamics between the victims and perpetrators have been found to impact exploitation risk in two described models [19]. Researchers described that older persons who experienced what they termed as "pure financial exploitation" (PFE) were generally financially or physically independent, as were their perpetrators. The described characteristics that increased susceptibility to financial exploitation included a variety of characteristics including these victims developing a false sense of trust along with a desire to protect the perpetrator. Other described schemes for financial exploitation include the development of a short-term romantic or sexual relationship with the perpetrator with financial assets as the "quid pro quo" requirement for the relationship to continue. In addition, the elderly victim often overestimated the skills or good intentions of the perpetrator or feared loss of independence and became enmeshed in circumstances that allowed the perpetrator to prey on this fear. Many victims were duped into being "charitable" and misled in their good intentions.

In comparison to victims of PFE, the described victims of "hybrid financial exploitation" (HFE) were typically physically or cognitively but not financially dependent on their perpetrator with their perpetrators generally financially dependent on the victim. Risks factors identified in this group of exploited older persons included co-occurring but unrelated financial exploitation and physical abuse in which the victim had sought to protect the dependent perpetrator in a "parent-child" relationship. This dependency in the perpetrator generally centered on mental illness or substance abuse issues. The authors concluded that PFE was more similar to crimes against society and HFE was more similar to family violence.

The many variables that contribute to financial exploitation of older persons in the United States include a cohort effect of unprecedented wealth, trust, and generosity in an unparalleled number of those aging into physical frailty and cognitive impairment, creating a concerning environment of vulnerability to abuse and financial exploitation. Patterns of abuse differ between gender and race, with females more likely to be victims of abuse overall and African-Americans more likely to be financially exploited. Social isolation, poor social support, and loneliness and

Table 1.1 Characteristics of vulnerability

Characteristics of vulnerability
Depression, bereavement, loneliness
Social isolation
Adult child living with elder
Dependence on another to provide care
Financially responsible for adult child, spouse, or trusted caregiver
Cognitively impaired
Physically impaired

(Adapted from Teaster [8])

depression also play a role. Perhaps the most confounding variable in the financial exploitation discussion is the effect of interpersonal dynamics within relationships that are frequently familial and lifelong. The enmeshed nature of these relationships makes the recognition, reporting, and the protection of those who are financially exploited particularly challenging (Table 1.1).

The National Impact of Elderly Financial Exploitation

In 2009, MetLife in conjunction with NCPEA and Virginia Tech published a groundbreaking study of elder financial exploitation that provided a comprehensive understanding about the extent and implications of all forms of elder financial abuse. This study, "Broken Trust: Elders, Family, and Finances," was the first large-scale study of its kind and used data from a number of resources [1] including news feed articles collected by the National APS via daily media releases tracked by Google or Yahoo search engines from April to June 2008; 12 electronic databases of academic journals containing primary literature from 1998 to 2008 with articles from organizational and trade literature; and the Promising Practice database maintained by NCEA. In a mere 3 months, the news feed articles revealed approximately $396,654,700 in losses from all forms of financial abuse which annualized to a staggering $1.5 billion per year. These losses represented figures reported in 60% of the articles. Extrapolating similar losses in the additional unreported cases, the authors estimated a potential yearly financial exploitation of closer to $2.6 billion per year. Business and industry-related losses resulted in the highest monetary losses to the victims, followed by Medicare and Medicaid fraud. Exploitation by individuals ranked last on the list. However, the perpetrators were most likely to be family, friends, neighbors, and caregivers (55%), with strangers (21%), financial professionals (18%), and Medicare/Medicaid fraud ranking lower in frequency.

Utilizing the similar methods, MetLife conducted a second study in 2010. Its published report, "Crimes of Occasion, Desperation, and Predation Against America's Elders," showed a 12% increase in financial exploitation in the 2 years that had elapsed from the initial study, with estimated losses now at $2.9 billion a year. In addition, there was a change in the manner of exploitation used, with a trend

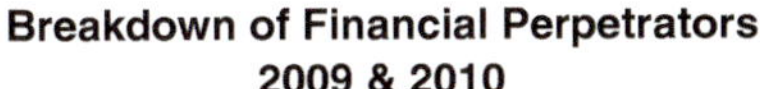

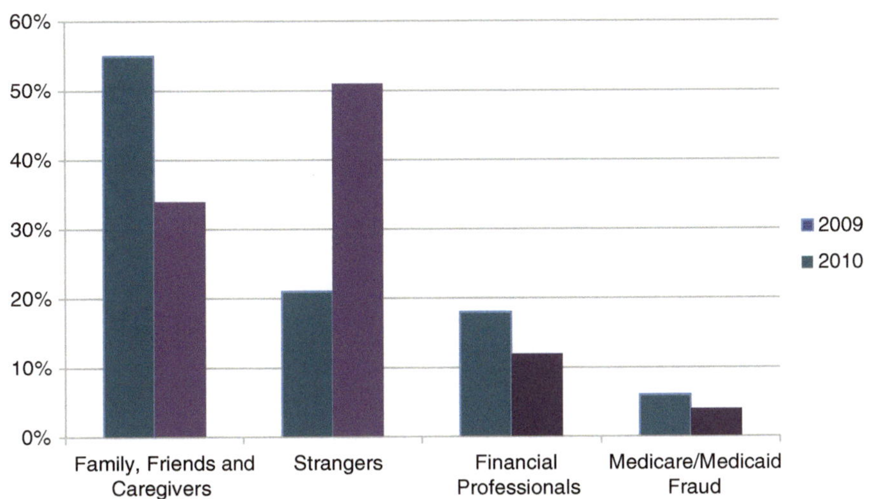

Fig. 1.3 Most common sources of financial abuse. (Adapted from Crimes of Occasion, Desperation, and Predation Against Americas Elderly [20])

toward increasing scams and confidence schemes. The perpetrators in these scenarios were more likely to be strangers (51%), with financial abuse by family, friends or neighbors (34%), business sector (12%), and finally Medicare or Medicaid fraud (4%). The profile of the perpetrator was largely male between the ages of 30 and 59 years. The ranking of monetary losses had likewise shifted, with Medicare or Medicaid fraud highest ($38,263,136), the business sector next ($6,219,496), family friends and neighbors third ($145,768), and fraud by strangers last ($95,156) [20] (Fig. 1.3).

The victims of this form of financial exploitation were more likely women (two-fold higher) between the ages of 80 and 89 who were reliant on others for health care, personal services, or home maintenance. "There existed a combination of tenuous, valued independence and observable vulnerability that merged in the lives of the victims to optimize opportunities for abuse by every type of perpetrator from closest family members to professional criminals." The 2010 data also showed a change in the types of crimes, with reports of phone scams, confidence schemes, and robberies rising from 9.5% to 28%. Crimes committed by family members decreased by half in this period, caregivers by one-third, and trusted individuals by two-thirds (Table 1.2).

Underscoring the vulnerability of these victims was the dramatic increase in the number of abusive and violent events occurring during the holidays, equally meted out by strangers and family. The often random, stranger-driven crimes were associated with a high level of brutality, characterized by a single event of severe beatings,

Table 1.2 Types of financial abuse

Crimes of occasion	Crimes of desperation	Crimes of predation
Theft	Misappropriation or misuse of money, property, or assets	Persuading an impaired elder person to change a will or insurance policy
Assault and robbery	Improper use of conservatorship, guardianship, or power of attorney	Improperly using the authority provided by a conservatorship, trust, etc.
Forcing or forging an older individual's signature on check	Denial to access of funds or preventing them from controlling their assets	Forced transfer of conservatorship
Taking money under false pretenses	Failure to repay loans	Telephone or internet scams
Identity theft	Living with another and not contributing to living expenses	Reverse mortgage scam
ATM or credit card use	Abusing joint signatory authority	Lottery scams
Carrying out unnecessary work or overcharging for work done	Using older person as guarantor of loan for personal benefits	Debt relief scam
Sweet heart scams	Cashing an older person's checks	Foreclosure rescue scam
	Overcharging for groceries or shopping for elder	Improper financial planning advice that does not meet the older individuals needs
	ATM or credit card use	Getting an older person to sign a will, contract, or power of attorney through deception, coercion, or undue influence
	Promising long-term care in exchange for money or property and then not providing the service	Exploitation by a financial institution employee
		Predatory lending

Adapted from Crimes of Occasion, Desperation, and Predation Against Americas Elderly [20]

rape, and murder. These events during the holiday study period rose to 28%, up from 12% in spring of 2010 and 3% as captured by the 2008 news feeds.

The Metlife review of the research from 2008 to 2010 published in academic peer reviewed journals across the social, medical, and legal disciplines showed four trends emerging in the financial exploitation literature. Studies showed an increase in both incidence and prevalence of such elderly exploitation [21–25]. Further definition of subpopulations of older persons at risk of financial exploitation was uncovered [16, 22, 26, 27] and insights on risks for financial abuse were made [28–31]. New measures or models to assess elder financial abuse were advanced [32–36]. In fact on further review, one in four vulnerable older persons was found at risk of financial exploitation and only a small portion of this abuse was being detected [37].

Certainly, the National Elder Mistreatment study (NEMS), a second large-scale study, confirms that abuse of the elderly is prevalent and increasing [21]. Using telephone survey of a nationally representative sample of elders by random digit dialing across geographic strata, of the 5777 respondents, the following results were reported: a 1 year prevalence of 5.2% of financial exploitation, 5.1% of potential neglect, 4.6% of emotional abuse, 1.6% of physical abuse, and 0.6% of sexual abuse. This was the first study to uncover the lead role that financial exploitation plays in the lives of its victims. Low social support, poor health, and required assistance with daily activities were predictors for such abuse.

This observation was likewise found in the 2011 New York State Elder Abuse Prevalence Study (NYSEAPS). Using the same methodology as NEMS, it documented a dramatic gap between the rate of elder abuse events and those reported and referred to the New York APS system. The reported cumulative prevalence of 46.2 per thousand for all forms of self-reported abuse has a true incidence that may be 24 times this number and 44 times the rate of self-reported cases of financial exploitation in New York [38].

Financial exploitation, along with other forms of elder abuse, has profound consequences. In a study conducted by Burnett et al. [39], mortality risk was assessed for five different types of abuse that were experienced by older individuals. This study, involving 1672 cases of substantiated elder abuse, found that the frequency of various type of abuse included caregiver neglect (34%), polyvictimization (31%), emotional abuse (19%), financial abuse (9%), and physical abuse (7%). Though the highest percentage of deaths were within a category of caregiver neglect (35%), financial abuse was linked to 28% of the cases, with polyvictimization following at 21%, emotional abuse at 17%, and physical abuse at 15%. This study highlighted the impact of financial exploitation not just from a monetary standpoint but also from a mortality standpoint.

Conclusions and Future Directions in Curbing Financial Exploitation in the Elderly

Described are the incidence of financial abuse in the elderly, groups at risk, and perpetrators of such crimes in the United States. Although the "typical" victim is female, age 80–89, and often cognitively or physically impaired, these statistics could mislead and belie simplicity to what is a complex and overarching societal problem. Subgroup analysis reveals numerous victims across gender and all racial groups but with differing patterns of abuse. While the impact of this abuse is staggering in financial terms (by some estimates close to $2.9 billion annually), it is also devastating in personal terms and raises societal concerns over the safety of the ill, infirm, and most vulnerable. In addition, the complexity of interpersonal dynamics that figures closely into many of these exploitation events often centers around issues of privacy, autonomy versus safety, and the potential for financial devastation. Drawing the ethical and legal line of what constitutes financial abuse and the interplay of advancing cognitive impairment may represent some of the more difficult debates, as many of the perpetrators are often close family members with long-established and patterned relationships with the elderly victim.

What is further concerning is the rising trend in victimization with financial exploitation up to 5.2% of elderly in the United States, especially as the country's baby boomers continue to age into frailty and dependence in large numbers, creating an even bigger risk pool. Changing trends in victimization with more financial fraud in Medicare and Medicaid and confidence schemes and scams call for continued surveillance and public education. Not just following trends but studying these emerging patterns of abuse with strong judicial backup at the federal and state levels may be crucial to the protection of the elderly victim. While more education and support at the level of the aging individual and public are needed, education of those who serve as protectors of the ill and debilitated (medical personnel, doctors, social workers, caseworkers, elderly advocates, law enforcement, and lawyers) requires judicial support.

Acknowledgments The current author of this chapter for this edition would like to acknowledge the significant contributions of the prior edition's authors of this chapter:

Ann T. Riggs, M.D., C.M.D.
Associate Professor of Medicine
Donald W. Reynolds, Department of Geriatrics
Paula M. Podrazik, M.D.
Associate Professor of Medicine
Donald W. Reynolds, Department of Geriatrics

References

1. Broken Trust: Elders, Family and Finances. Metlife Study, March 2009. Available from: http://www.metlife.com/assets/cao/nmi/publications/studies/nmi-study-broken-trust-elders-family-finances.pdf.
2. Aging into the 21st Century. Administration on Aging; modified 2011. Available from: http://www.aoa.gov/AoARoot/Aging_Statistics/future-growth/aging/21/health.aspx.
3. Sixty-five plus in the United States. U.S. Census Bureau Statistical Brief; 1995 May. Available from: http://www.census.gov/populaton/socdemo/statbriefs/agebrief.html.
4. Elder Maltreatment: Definition. Centers for Disease Control; 2010. Available from http://www.cdc.gov/ViolencePrevention/eldermaltreatment/definitions.html.
5. National Center on Elder Abuse; 1998. Available from:http://www.ncea.aoa.gov/Main_SiteFAQ/Basics/Types_Of_Abuse.aspx.
6. Older Americans Act and Aging Network. Section 102,18 A. Exploitation Definition. Administration on Aging; modified 2012.
7. The National Elder Abuse Incidence study: Prepared for The Administration for Children and Families and The Administration on Aging in The U.S. Department of Health and Human Services. Available from: http://www.aoa.gov/aoARoot/AOA_Programs/Elder_Rights/Elder_Abuse.
8. Teaster TB. A response to the abuse of vulnerable adults; The 2000 Survey of State Adult Protective Services; 2000. Available from: http://www.nceaao.gov/resources/publications/docs/aps.reportto30703.pdf.

9. Teaster TB, et al. Abuse of Adults 60 Years of Age or Older Report to the National Center on Elder Abuse, Administration on Aging Washington DC; 2004. The 2004 Survey of adult Protective Services. Available from: http://www.ncea.aoa.gov/ncearoot/main_site/pdf/2-14-06%20FINAL%2060+REPORT.pdf.
10. Lauman EO. Elder mistreatment in the United States: prevalence estimates from a nationally representative study. J Gerontol Soc Sci. 2008;63B(4):S248–54.
11. Federal Trade Commission. (2019, October 18). Protecting Older Consumers 2018–2019: A Report of the Federal Trade Commission. Retrieved from https://www.ftc.gov/system/files/documents/reports/protecting-older-consumers-2018-2019-report-federal-trade-commission/p144401_protecting_older_consumers_2019_1.pdf
12. Elder justice and protection: Stopping the financial Abuse. Hearing before the Subcommittee on Aging; 2003 October. Available from: http:www.gpo.gov/fdsys/pkg/CHRG-108shrg90305/html/CHRG-108shrg90305.htm
13. Hafemeister TL. Financial exploitation in domestic situations. In: Richard JB, Wallace RB, editors. Elder mistreatment: abuse, neglect, and exploitation in ageing America. Washington D.C.: The National Academies Press; 2003. p. 88–103.
14. Malks B, Buckmaster J, Cunningham L. Combating elder financial abuse: a multi-disciplinary approach to a growing problem. J Elder Abuse Neglect. 2003;15:55–75.
15. Choi NG, Mayer J. Elder abuse, neglect, and exploitation risk factors and prevention strategies. J Gerontol Soc Work. 2000;33(2):5–25.
16. Beach SR. Financial exploitation and psychological mistreatment among older adults: differences between African Americans and Non-African Americans in a population–based survey. The Gerontologist. 2010;50(6, 744)
17. Okonkwo O, et al. Cognitive correlates of financial abilities in mild cognitive impairment. J Am Geriatr Soc. 2006;4(11):1745–50.
18. Denburg NL, et al. The orbitofrontal cortex, real-world decision making, and normal aging. Ann N Y Acad Sci. 2007;1121:480–98.
19. Jackson SL, Haefemeister TL. Risk factors associated with elder abuse: the importance of differentiating by type for elder maltreatment. Violence Vict. 2011;26:738.
20. Crimes of occasion, desperation, and predation against Americas elderly. Metlife Study of Financial Abuse. 2011;1–25.
21. Aceierno R. Prevalence and correlates of emotional, physical, sexual, and financial abuse and potential neglect in the United States: the National Elder Mistreatment Study. Am J Public Health. 2010;100:202–97.
22. Christiansen MA. Unconscionable: financial exploitation of elderly persons with dementia. Marquette Elder's Advisor. 2008;2:383–416.
23. Garre-Olmo J, Planas-Pujol X, Lopez-Pousa S, Juvinya D, Vila A, et al. Prevalence and risk factors of suspected elder abuse subtypes in people aged 75 and older. J Am Geriatr Soc. 2009;57:815–22.
24. Guardianships: Cases of financial exploitation, neglect, and abuse of seniors (GAO-10-1046). Washington, D.C.: United States Government Accountability Office. General Accountability Office, 2009 September.
25. Lowenstein A, Eisikovits Z, Band-Winterstein T, Enosh G. Is elder abuse and neglect asocial phenomenon? Data from the First National Prevalence Survey in Israel. J Elder Abuse Neglect. 2009;21:253–77.
26. Bond JB Jr, Cuddy R, Dixon GL, Duncan KA, Smith D. The financial abuse of mentally incompetent older adults: a Canadian study. J Elder Abuse Neglect. 1999;11(4):23–38.
27. Lee HY, Eaton CK. Financial abuse in elderly Korean immigrants: mixed analysis of the role of culture on perception and help-seeking intention. J Gerontol Social Work. 2009;52(5):463–88.
28. Bendix J. Exploiting the elderly. RN. 2009;72(3):42–6.
29. Black JA. The not-so-golden years: power of attorney, elder abuse, and why our laws are failing a vulnerable population. St John's Law Rev. 2008;82:289–314.

30. Buzgova R, Ivanova K. Elder abuse and mistreatment in residential settings. Nurs Ethics. 2009;16(1):110–26.
31. Phillips LR, Guo G. Mistreatment in assisted living facilities: complaints, substantiations, and risk factors. The Gerontologist. 2011:1–11. https://doi.org/10.1093/geront/gnq122.
32. Anthony EK, Lehning AJ, Austin MJ, Peck MD. Assessing elder mistreatment: Instrument development and implications for adult protective services. J Gerontologic Social Work. 2009;52(8):815–36, lect 14(2/3),9–31.
33. Conrad KJ, Iris M, Ridings JW, Langley K, Wilber KH. Self-report measure of financial exploitation of older adults. The Gerontologist. 2010;50(6):758–73.
34. Goergen T, Beaulieu M. Criminological theory and elder abuse research — fruitful relationship or worlds apart. Ageing Int. 2010;35:185–201.
35. Hawes C, Kimbell AM. Detecting, addressing, and preventing elder abuse in residential care facilities. Report to the National Institute of Justice, US Dept. of Justice. (2010) Retrieved January 6, 2020 from www.ncjrs.gov/pdffiles1/nij/grants/229299.pdf.
36. Pinske DM, McFarland K, Pachana NK. Exploitation in older adults: social vulnerability and personal competence factors. J Appl Gerontol. 2010;29(6):740–61.
37. Cooper C, Selwood A, Livingston G. The prevalence of elder abuse and neglect: a systematic review. Age Ageing. 2008;37(2):151–60.
38. Lifespan of Greater Rochester Under the Radar: New York Elder Abuse Prevalence Study. Self-Reported Prevalence and Documented Case Surveys. Final Report Executive Summary, 2011. Available from: http://www.nyselderabuse.org/prevalence-study.html.
39. Burnett J, Jackson SL, Sinha AK, Aschenbrenner AR, Murphy KP, Xia R, Diamond PM. Five-year all-cause mortality rates across five categories of substantiated elder abuse occurring in the community. J Elder Abuse Negl. 2016;28(2):59–75. https://doi.org/10.1080/08946566.2016.1142920.

Chapter 2
One Piece of the Puzzle – Financial Exploitation and Elder Abuse

Sherif Soliman and Jason Beaman

Introduction

True and current estimates of elder financial abuse are not known. A sentinel study in this arena is the 2009 MetLife Broken Trust study. This study estimates that the annual financial loss by senior citizens is 2.6 billion dollars [1]. It affects a wide array of victims and is committed by a diverse group of perpetrators ranging from close family members to professional con artists. In a 2011 follow-up study, MetLife found that the number had risen to 2.9 billion dollars [2]. Even that higher number is likely an underestimate since it is based on a survey of cases reported in the media. In fact, a 2015 survey by True Link Financial, a firm that specializes in financial products designed to protect elder investors, estimates the loss at 36.48 billion dollars a year [3].

The National Center on Elder Abuse defines elder financial abuse broadly as "theft, fraud, misuse or neglect of authority, and use of undue influence as a lever to gain control over an older person's money or property" [4]. This type of abuse takes many forms, including "cashing an older person's checks without authorization or permission; forging an older person's signature; misusing or stealing an older person's money or possessions; coercing or deceiving an older person into signing any document; and the improper use of conservatorship, guardianship, or power of attorney" [4]. Elder financial abuse can co-occur in the context of other forms of abuse such as physical abuse (hybrid financial abuse) or by itself (pure financial abuse). Hybrid financial abuse differs from pure financial abuse by methods used,

S. Soliman (✉)
Forensic and Geriatric Psychiatry, Atrium Health, Charlotte, NC, USA

J. Beaman
Department of Psychiatry and Behavioral Sciences, Oklahoma State University Center for Health Sciences, Tulsa, OK, USA

R. M. Factora (ed.), *Aging and Money*,
https://doi.org/10.1007/978-3-030-67565-3_2

offender profile, and victim profile. Thus, elder financial abuse is both one piece of the broader puzzle of elder abuse and a puzzle onto itself.

In addition to elder financial abuse, there are four other types of elder abuse: physical abuse, emotional abuse, sexual abuse, and neglect (including self-neglect). Physical abuse refers to the "use of physical force that may result in bodily injury, physical pain, or impairment" [4]. Emotional abuse is "the infliction of pain, anguish, or distress through verbal or nonverbal acts" [4]. Sexual abuse is "nonconsensual sexual contact of any kind with an elderly person" [4]. Neglect is the "refusal or failure to fulfill any part of a caregiver's obligation or duty to an elder" [4].

Elder financial abuse has been called the crime of the twenty-first century. The costs are staggering and the effect on victims is often devastating. Victims are often left destitute and homeless. They lose the liberty to manage their own affairs because they require guardianship to stop the financial abuse and protect them against further abuse. Elder financial abuse is expected to continue to increase secondary to a perfect storm of demographic, economic, and technological factors and physical or cognitive factors. First, the population of adults over 60 years of age increased 35% from 52.5 million to 70.8 million from 2007 to 2017. Projections for 2040 indicate that the number of individuals over the age of 85 will increase from 6.5 million in 2017 to 14.4 million [5]. Second, older individuals have more wealth to be exploited. According to Forbes Magazine, the Silent Generation (individuals born between 1925 and 1942) experienced the largest growth in wealth over all other age groups. This cohort has 1.3 times the amount of Boomers (1944 and 1964), twice the amount of Generation X (1965 and 1979), and 23 times the wealth of Generation Y (also known as Millennials, 1980–1994) [6]. Third, technological advances such as online banking and stock trading have made money management more complex and have made perpetrating large-scale fraud easier. Fourth, elderly victims often have physical or cognitive limitations that render them both more dependent on others and less able to critically evaluate potential scams.

This chapter will discuss elder financial abuse as part of the broader problem of elder abuse. It will outline the scope of the problem of elder financial abuse, the types of financial abuse, victim profiles, and perpetrator profiles. It will discuss undue influence as a unique mechanism of elder financial abuse. It will offer recommendations for a multidisciplinary approach to preventing and combatting elder financial abuse.

Scope of the Problem

Elder abuse in general often goes unreported. One study found that for every case that is reported, 24 are not [7]. This study found that this was much higher for financial abuse, a ratio of 43.9 cases for every one reported [5]. Also, there is variability in data collection, which is believed to contribute to the large gap between reported and actual cases [7].

Elder financial abuse goes unreported for several reasons. Victims often fear reporting because of safety concerns. They may be unaware that they are being exploited because of lack of control over their finances. Some victims believe that the perpetrators are actually acting in their best interest. Victims do not report the abuse out of embarrassment. Finally, some victims don't report because they feel loyalty toward the perpetrator, especially when the perpetrator is a close family member.

With these caveats, studies have varied in their estimates of the prevalence. The prevalence is listed as 5.2% [8], 1.3% [9], and 1.4% [10]. Rates are different within cultural groups. The Latino population has rates as high as 16.7% [11]. Non-white persons have an odds ratio of 1.29 for financial mistreatment [8]. Financial abuse often co-occurs with other types of elder abuse. One study suggested a rate as high as 21% of multiple types of abuse [12].

The National Elder Abuse Incidence Study of 1998 estimated that there were 449,924 cases of elder abuse (551,011 including self-neglect) [11]. Of the confirmed cases that they reviewed, 30.2% were of elder financial abuse [11]. A subsequent survey by the National Center on Elder Abuse found that Adult Protective Services in 2004 found that there were 565,467 cases of elder and vulnerable adult abuse reported to state Adult Protective Services agencies, a 19% increase from the 2000 survey [13]. Of these reports, 253,426 concerned adults aged 60 and older. Among the cases investigated by Adult Protective Services agencies, 20.8% were cases of elder financial abuse. Self-neglect was the most common form of elder abuse, accounting for 26.7% of investigated cases followed by caregiver neglect (23.7%), emotional abuse (13.6%), physical abuse (12.5%), and sexual abuse (0.7%). Looking at substantiated cases of elder abuse yields a largely similar picture: self-neglect (37.2%), caregiver neglect (20.4%), emotional abuse (14.8%), financial abuse (14.7%), physical abuse (10.7%), and sexual abuse (1%) [13].

Pure Financial Abuse Versus Hybrid Financial Abuse

Pure financial abuse is the abuse that occurs in the absence of other forms of elder abuse. This phenomenon differs significantly from hybrid financial abuse, which occurs concurrently with other forms of elder abuse, such as physical or emotional abuse.

In a 2011 report to the US Department of Justice, Jackson and Hafmeister interviewed 71 elderly victims of financial exploitation in Virginia and the Adult Protective Services worker for each victim in order to examine financial exploitation of the elderly compared to other forms of elder abuse [14]. One portion of the study compared victims and perpetrators of pure financial abuse to those of hybrid financial abuse. Pure financial abuse is more likely to be perpetrated by nonfamily members (compared to hybrid financial abuse). Compared with victims of hybrid financial abuse, these victims tend to live alone, are more financially and physically independent, are younger in age, and have less cognitive and communication difficulties. Hybrid financial abuse is usually perpetrated by family members or caregivers [14]. The victims tend to be older, more physically and financially dependent, more impaired, more isolated, and in poorer health [14]. The victims often live with the perpetrators and perceive the perpetrators as being supportive [14]. The perpetrators were unemployed and financially dependent on the victims [14].

Types of Elder Financial Abuse

Elder financial abuse can be categorized into three types based upon the context of the abuse: occasion, desperation, and predation [2]. Crimes of occasion occur when a perpetrator, who otherwise would not commit financial exploitation, is placed in a situation where he/she has the opportunity to commit financial abuse. Crimes of desperation are acts of financial abuse because the perpetrator is in dire financial straits and will do anything to obtain money. Crimes of predation, as the name implies, are acts of abuse in which the perpetrator actively seeks out vulnerable victims. Some instances of elder financial abuse have elements of more than one type.

The prototypical crime of occasion occurs when a family member or trusted friend exploits a senior relative who has recently become vulnerable by virtue of illness, loss, or isolation. The "occasion" of the victim's vulnerability can create opportunities for would-be perpetrators in unusual ways. When 83-year-old Anna Mae Franklin discovered that her recently widowed brother, Arthur Cropsey [91], suffered from Alzheimer's disease, she immediately moved him into her home and helped manage his finances using a power of attorney. Unbeknownst to her, she created an opportunity for financial abuse. She discovered that her daughter had been spending large amounts of his money. She took the painful step of reporting her daughter, who was subsequently court ordered to pay back $40,000 [15].

William Shakespeare's admonition, "Tempt not a desperate man," is as true today as it was in 1595 [16]. Desperation can turn caring family members into perpetrators of financial abuse who drain the assets of their parents and grandparents. Crimes of desperation are often committed by family members and can take many forms such as borrowing excessive amounts of money and not returning it, committing fraud, or extorting money with threats. The common theme in this category is that the crime would not otherwise be committed aside from circumstances of the perpetrator. These crimes often involve escalating steps of exploitation. It may start with borrowing money with honest intentions and escalate as the perpetrator becomes more desperate.

Not surprisingly, perpetrators of crimes of desperation tend to be financially dependent on the elder and are more likely to be addicted to drugs or alcohol. More men than women commit crimes of desperation [2]. The perpetrator may rationalize by believing that they are due compensation for the care they provide. This can facilitate the crime to continue as long as they are involved in the victim's life.

Predation is the act of seeking out the victim intentionally to form a relationship, which will allow the abuse. This involves seeking out a new romantic or financial relationship with the specific intent of exploiting the elder for financial gain. The perpetrators are usually strangers and can be professional con artists. This crime can be perpetrated by an unscrupulous professional who seek these victims out. These professionals have financial access to the elders, including stockbrokers, financial advisors, and insurance agents, among others. There have been reports of religious personalities and political parties also exploiting the elderly. However, it is important to note that this does not usually involve the formation of a relationship for that purpose [2].

Unfortunately, as technology has advanced and finances have become more complex, con artists have found virtually limitless ways to prey upon their victims.

The National Council on Aging provides a list of the top ten scams targeting seniors [17]. The most common was healthcare fraud. Perpetrators pose as healthcare providers and offer fraudulent services in makeshift "clinics." They then bill Medicare for these fraudulent services. Other common scams include reverse mortgage fraud, telemarketing fraud, and fraudulent investments. One particularly cruel hoax is the "grandparent scam." The perpetrator calls and immediately greets the victim as "grandma" or "grandpa." They then tell the victim that they are in trouble and need money wired immediately. They beg the unsuspecting victim not to tell their parents.

The faces of elder financial abuse are diverse and expanding. The different forms of elder financial abuse occur in unique settings, by a wide variety of perpetrators, and against a wide array of seniors. Table 2.1 summarizes the different signs of

Table 2.1 Signs of potential financial exploitation by category [11, 18]

Type	Signs
Social	Stranger suddenly befriends elder and becomes close very quickly Previously uninvolved family members suddenly become involved and claim rights to the elder's funds The elder becomes isolated from prior contacts
Medical	Elder appears to be receiving substandard care despite adequate resources Elder suddenly can no longer afford medications and copays Elder displays other signs of abuse and neglect such as dehydration, bruising, bedsores, malnutrition Caregiver refuses to allow elder to be interviewed alone Elder depressed and helpless A new physician is sought out to complete an evaluation for guardianship by the caregiver
Financial	Unexplained withdrawals of large sums of money Previously independent elder is accompanied to financial institutions Checks written by elder to "cash" or to single individual for large sums of money Change of beneficiary on elder's accounts Discovery that elder's signature has been forged Sudden addition of previously uninvolved person to elder's bank or credit card accounts
Legal	Unexplained changes in longstanding will or trust Changes in will procured by a third party New attorney retained by a third party to change the elder's will Elder brought to the attorney's office by the beneficiary of changes to the elder's will

financial exploitation that may be encountered. Whether the crime is one of occasion, desperation, or predation, it exacts a devastating toll on its victims. Victims become hurt, ashamed, depressed, and sometimes destitute.

Victims and Perpetrators

Victim and perpetrator profiles vary based upon the type of elder abuse and the context in which it occurs (domestic vs. institutional). We will begin by reviewing briefly the common characteristics of victims and perpetrators of elder abuse in general and then discuss the characteristics of financial exploitation victims and perpetrators. In general, victims and perpetrators of hybrid financial exploitation more closely resemble those of elder abuse in general. Pure financial exploitation is a distinct entity in that it is committed by a different group of perpetrators, affects a relatively higher functioning group of victims, and is more likely committed by professional con artists.

Victims

In the 2004 Survey of Adult Protective Services, the majority of victims by sex were female (65.7%). By age, most victims were above 80 (42.8%). By race, most victims were Caucasian (77.1%). By location, the majority of abuse occurred in domestic settings (89.3%) [13].

While the elderly as a group are at increased risk for financial abuse, there are unique risk factors that place victims at especially high risk. They can be divided into physical, psychiatric, and social risk factors. Physical risk factors include advanced age (75 or older), limited mobility, sensory impairment, frailty, and organic brain damage [18]. Psychiatric risk factors include dementia, mental illness, especially depression, and personality disorders that cause isolation (avoidant and schizoid) [18]. Social risk factors include recent loss of spouse, female gender, living alone, living with the suspected perpetrator, and owning a home [18].

Victim profiles differ based upon the type of financial abuse. Victims of pure financial exploitation tend to be higher functioning, have less cognitive impairment, live alone, have no children, have no communication problems, and have a good relationship with the perpetrator [14]. In contrast, victims of hybrid financial abuse tend to be older, are dependent on the perpetrator, have more cognitive impairment, be isolated, be widowed, live with the perpetrator, and be in poorer health. In addition, victims of hybrid financial abuse were likely to have a longer history of abuse and have a childhood history of abuse compared to victims of pure financial abuse [14].

Perpetrators

In the 2004 Survey of Adult Protective Services, perpetrators were slightly more likely to be female (52.7%). The most frequent perpetrators of elder abuse were adult children (32.6%). More than two-thirds of perpetrators were under age 60 (75.1%) [13].

There are some differences between male and female perpetrators and between perpetrators of different types of financial abuse. Approximately 60% of perpetrators are males between the ages of 30 and 59 [2]. Male perpetrators have such traits as antisocial personality disorder, being caregivers, living with the victim, being economically dependent on the victim, and have a history of mental illness or substance abuse [18]. They also themselves have health problems [18].

Most female perpetrators are between the ages of 30 and 49 [2]. Other characteristics of female perpetrators include having a caregiving relationship with the victim and instilling a sense of helplessness and dependency. Female perpetrators will often isolate the victim from family and friends, often acting as a protector. Female perpetrators also have a history of multiple unstable relationships and will falsify personal information (such as credentials or roles) [18]. They are opportunistic and psychologically dysfunctional [18]. They exhibit predatory behavior and like males, females can also have antisocial personality traits. Female perpetrators will methodically identify victims that they can exert total control over [18]. This control will then be used to implement the exploitation.

Hybrid financial abuse is more likely to be perpetrated by parasitic abusers (financially dependent on the victim) who are related to the victim and unemployed [14]. In contrast, perpetrators of pure financial exploitation are more likely to be nonrelatives, not parasitic, and less likely to have a history of domestic violence [14].

Undue Influence and the Psychodynamics of Exploitation

One of the most important mechanisms used to commit elder financial abuse is undue influence. Undue influence is "any act of persuasion that overcomes the free will and judgment of another" [19]. Undue influence occurs when a vulnerable person's will is subjugated to the desires of another person. The doctrine of undue influence has typically been applied to wills. However, it is also applied to inter vivos gifts or gifts given while the elder is living.

Undue influence begins with a susceptible victim. As discussed above, indicators of victim susceptibility include physical or mental illness, dementia, recent loss, or isolation. It should be noted that many of the traits often co-occur (such as the wife who recently lost her husband and is now isolated). The psychological process of exerting undue influence upon another has been likened to other processes of exploitation. These include intimate partner violence and the process of indoctrination used by cults.

Psychologist Margaret Singer has identified six psychological mechanisms used by perpetrators of undue influence: isolation, creating a siege mentality, fostering dependence, creating a sense of powerlessness, creating fear and vulnerability, and keeping the target unaware [20]. Similar psychological factors have been descried in domestic violence and elder abuse.

Isolation is one of the most significant risk factors for elder financial exploitation. Many victims of elder abuse are already isolated, making them more vulnerable to the advances of the perpetrator. Methods of isolation include limiting visits, blocking telephone calls and other communication, and using deception to turn the victim against family and friends. The perpetrator may extend that isolation by convincing or compelling the victim to switch to new physicians, attorneys, or financial planners. This also makes it less likely that the abuse will be detected because the new providers are less familiar with the victim, his/her health status, and his/her previously expressed wishes with regard to financial management and estate planning. Perpetrators create a "siege mentality" by portraying the outside world as a dangerous place and portraying themselves as protectors. They may falsely accuse family members or trusted friends of trying to harm or take advantage of the elder. They foster a sense of powerlessness, fear, and vulnerability by convincing the elder that he/she is not capable of managing their affairs alone and that harm would befall them but for the perpetrator's "help." They foster a sense of dependence by gradually seizing control of the victim's assets, and in many cases, the victim's ability to make even basic decisions. The sense of dependence is deepened because the perpetrator often indoctrinates the victim with exaggerated or fabricated claims of how dangerous it would be for the victim to manage his/her own affairs. Finally, they necessarily keep the target unaware throughout this process.

While we often think of victims of elder abuse as frail and powerless, anyone can become a victim of elder abuse. On March 2, 2011, famed actor Mickey Rooney (then 90) testified before the Senate Select Committee on Aging about his longstanding elder abuse [21]. He alleged that his stepson and stepdaughter neglected him, emotionally abused him, and financially exploited him. In his testimony, he described several of the psychological aspects of elder abuse and exploitation:

> What other people see as generosity may, in reality, be the exploitation, manipulation, and sadly, emotional blackmail of older, more vulnerable members of the American public. I know because it happened to me. My money was taken and misused. When I asked for information, I was told that I couldn't have any of my own information. I was told it was "for my own good" and that "it was none of my business." I was literally left powerless. You can be in control of your life one minute and in the next minute, you have absolutely no control. Sometimes this happens quickly, but other times it is very gradual. You wonder when it truly began. In my case, I was eventually and completely stripped of the ability to make even the most basic decisions in my own life [21].

Mickey Rooney described feeling powerless, being told that he couldn't manage his own affairs, and not realizing when he lost control of his basic decision-making.

There are aspects of relationships, the so-called "red flags," that can give rise to undue influence. These red flags include secluding, providing attention, acceptance, and approval, fostering regression and dependence, depriving the victim of physical and mental privacy, indoctrination, reinforcing the new beliefs and behaviors, and disparaging independent thought [22].

Undue influence is a special mechanism for perpetrating elder financial abuse and a basis for overturning wills. However, the elements of undue influence are not unique and are often present in abusive relationships in general.

Table 2.2 summarizes many of the techniques used by perpetrators in their efforts to take advantage of vulnerable older persons. A greater discussion of this topic is addressed in Chap. 4.

Table 2.2 The Perpetrator's Playbook: Psychology of Exploitation and Undue Influence [20]

Technique	Tactics	Examples
Isolation	Depriving person of physical and mental space Discouraging communication Physically secluding Socially secluding	Moving to new area Preventing mail from being viewed Preventing telephone calls Preventing participation in social groups such as clubs or religious groups
Creating a "siege mentality"	Portraying world as dangerous Financial fears Describing crime in area around elder	Suggesting that family and friends are trying to steal money "Exposing" trusted professionals as attempting to con the elder Continuously discussing crimes in area Discussing physical dangers such as car accidents and falls
Creating dependence	Emphasizing elder's physical impairments Emphasizing intellectual deficits Emphasizing emotional vulnerabilities	Not allowing elder to do previous tasks such as basic housework Discouraging walks and other exercise Discouraging elder from doing his/her finances
Fostering powerlessness	Taking over prior roles	Doing everything for elder such as shopping, bills, housework
Creating fear and vulnerability	Casting previously trusted family members and others as villains	Telling the elder he/she has already been victim of theft from family or professionals Emphasizing dangers
Keeping target unaware	Cutting off communication	Not telling elder when family calls Not delivering letters or e-mails Not delivering bills that the elder would recognize as bogus

Combatting Elder Financial Abuse as Part of an Overall Strategy Against Elder Abuse

Fighting elder financial abuse requires a multimodal strategy that focuses on prevention, detection, protection, and deterrence. Prevention of elder financial abuse is accomplished by educating seniors about elder financial abuse, about common scams targeting the elderly, and resources in the community to combat elder financial abuse. In addition, educating caregivers, physicians, attorneys, and financial professionals about the signs of elder financial abuse can help detect financial abuse in the early stages and thereby mitigate the damage. It is also important to educate professionals about mandatory reporting requirements as misconceptions about reporting requirements often cause professionals to fail to report suspected abuse.

Detection

A multidisciplinary approach to the detection of elder financial abuse is required. The key professionals involved are caregivers, Adult Protective Services workers, physicians and other healthcare professionals, attorneys, and financial professionals. The indicators of financial abuse can be categorized into subsets pertinent to each discipline.

The Elder Abuse Incidence Study found that most elder abuse by others was reported by family members (20%), followed by hospitals (17.3%), police (11.3%), in-home caregivers (9.6%), friends or neighbors (9.1%), victims (8.8%), physicians and nurses (8.4%), out-of-home service providers (5.2%), and banks (0.4%). The top three reporters of financial exploitation were friends and neighbors (15%), hospitals (14.2%), and family members (14%) [11].

Caregivers (especially family members) are in an ideal position to notice if the elder suddenly befriends a new person and begins to transfer significant sums of money to that person. In fact, the majority of reports of elder abuse are already made by family members.

Healthcare professionals are often an early line of defense because the elderly often have frequent contact with them. Physical abuse or neglect is likely to be more apparent to the healthcare provider than financial exploitation, so it is important for providers to consider financial exploitation whenever they identify other forms of elder abuse. Healthcare providers should suspect elder financial abuse if their patient appears to be living substantially below their means, if the caregiver is managing the elder's funds but not providing basic necessities, if the elder has a sudden apparent decline in socioeconomic status, and if the caregiver insists on being present during every aspect of the examination though the senior appears capable of providing information. Physicians and other healthcare professionals may consider utilizing a standardized instrument to detect elder abuse, many of which contain questions relevant to financial abuse [23].

Attorneys should be educated about issues of financial exploitation and undue influence as they pertain to the preparation of wills, trusts, and powers of attorney. Changes in longstanding testamentary privileges, unnatural provisions added to a will, or changes in wills that are procured by a third party (especially if that party benefits from the change) should arouse suspicion. Changes in multiple instruments at the same time (e.g., will and power of attorney) should arouse suspicion that effective control of a victim's affairs is being transferred.

Financial professionals can also play a key role in detecting elder financial abuse. Suspicion should be aroused by unnatural changes in beneficiaries on accounts such as removing longstanding beneficiaries in favor of new people, changes in the elder's spending patterns, and suddenly liquidating accounts. The Investor Protection Trust has published a checklist and pocket guide for investment professionals to help them identify suspected cases of financial exploitation [24].

Protection

Once elder abuse has been detected, protection of the victim is the first priority. Adult Protective Services can investigate the alleged abuse and arrange for the victim to be removed immediately if there is imminent danger to the victim. In the case of physical abuse, sexual abuse, or neglect, the victim almost always requires immediate medical attention. Once abuse is uncovered and the victim is safe, it is important to take legal steps to restrict the perpetrator's access to the victim's funds. The specific steps will depend upon the legal mechanisms the perpetrator used to gain access to the victim. For example, if the perpetrator has obtained guardianship over the victim, the court of jurisdiction will need to be informed of the abuse and a petition filed to remove the guardian. A new guardian may be needed if the victim does indeed require guardianship. The next step is protecting the senior from further abuse. The specific interventions required will depend upon the elder's capacities, impairments, and needs. They will also depend upon the type of abuse suffered and the identity of the perpetrator.

Prosecuting cases of elder abuse is important in order to obtain justice for the victims, collect restitution (often not possible because abusers have spent the money and have few assets), and deter further abuse. Many con artists prey upon the elderly precisely because they believe the victims would make poor witnesses in court.

Conclusion

Financial exploitation is part of the growing problem of elder abuse. It can occur alone or in conjunction with other forms of elder abuse. It consists of three categories: crimes of occasion, crimes of desperation, and crimes of predation. The faces of elder financial abuse, both perpetrators and victims, vary significantly based upon whether the financial abuse occurs alone or with other forms of abuse. The psychodynamics of elder financial abuse, like other forms of abuse, are marked by isolation, creating a "siege mentality," creating a sense of fear and vulnerability, creating powerlessness, fostering dependence, and keeping the victim unaware.

Combatting elder financial abuse must be part of the broader strategy of fighting elder abuse. It will require a multidisciplinary approach. Healthcare professionals, attorneys, and financial professionals can all be instrumental in detecting, reporting, and stopping abuse. Combatting the crime of the twenty-first century must be our top priority. Our parents and grandparents deserve no less.

References

1. Broken Trust: Elders, Family, and Finances. A study on elder financial abuse prevention. Published online march 2009. https://www.giaging.org/documents/mmi-study-broken-trust-elders-family-finances.pdf. Accessed May 30 2020.
2. The MetLife study of elder financial abuse: crimes of occasion, desperation, and predation against America's elders. 2011. Available from: http://www.metlife.com/assets/cao/mmi/publications/studies/2011/mmi-elder-financial-abuse.pdf.
3. The True Link Report on Elder Financial Abuse 2015. https://d1qqb8hu7huvwj.cloudfront.net/uploads/2019/07/True-Link-Report-On-Elder-Financial-Abuse-012815.pdf. Accessed July 3 2020.
4. Red Flags of Abuse. National Center on Elder Abuse. Available from: https://ncea.acl.gov/NCEA/media/docs/Red-Flags-of-Elder-Abuse-English.pdf. Accessed May 30 2020
5. 2018 Older Americans Profile. Administration for Community Living. Published online 2018. https://acl.gov/sites/default/files/Aging%20and%20Disability%20in%20America/2018OlderAmericansProfile.pdf. Accessed May 30 2020.
6. Howe N. The Graying of wealth. Forbes. March 16, 2018. https://www.forbes.com/sites/neilhowe/2018/03/16/the-graying-of-wealth/.
7. Under the Radar: New York State Elder Abuse Prevalence Study. Lifespan of Greater Rochester, Inc., Weill Cornell Medical Center of Cornell University, New York City Department for the Aging. May 2011. https://ocfs.ny.gov/main/reports/Under%20the%20Radar%2005%2012%2011%20final%20report.pdf.
8. Aciemo R. Prevalence and correlates of emotional, physical, sexual, and financial abuse and potential neglect in the United States: the national elder mistreatment study. Am J Public Health. 2010;100(2):292–7.
9. Cooper C. The prevalence of elder abuse and neglect: a systematic review. Age Ageing. 2008;37:151–60.
10. Comi HC. Elder abuse in the community. J Am Geriatr Soc. 1998;46(7):885–8.
11. Tatara T, Kuzmeskus LB, Duckhorn E, Bivens L, Thomas C, Gertig J, Jay K, Hartley A. September 1998. The National Elder Abuse Incidence Study. https://acl.gov/sites/default/files/programs/2016-09/ABuseReport_Full.pdf.
12. DeLiema M. Determining prevalence and correlates of elder abuse using promotores: low-income immigrant Latinos report high rates of abuse and neglect. J Am Geriatric Soc. 2012;60(7):1333–9.
13. The National Committee for the Prevention of Elder Abuse and The National Adult Protective Services Association. The 2004 survey of state adult protective services: abuse of adults 60 years of age and older. February 2006. Available from: http://www.ncea.aoa.gov/ncearoot/main_site/pdf/2-14-06%20final%2060+report.pdf.

14. Jackson SL, Hafemeister TL. Financial abuse of elderly people vs. other forms of elder abuse: assessing their dynamics, risk factors, and society's response. Presented to the National Institute of Justice, U.S. Department of Justice, August 2010. Available from: https://www.ncjrs.gov/pdffiles1/nij/grants/233613.pdf.
15. Donahue K. One woman's story of elder financial abuse. Marketplace: your money. American Public Media. Aired November 16, 2012. Available from: https://www.marketplace.org/2012/11/16/one-womans-story-elder-financial-abuse/. Accessed May 31 2020.
16. Shakespeare W, Durband A. *Romeo and Juliet*. Woodbury: Barron's. Act 5, Scene 3, Page 3. 1985.
17. National Council on Aging. The top ten scams targeting seniors. Available at: http://www.ncoa.org/enhance-economic-security/economic-security-Initiative/savvy-saving-seniors/top-10-scams-targeting.html. Accessed May 31 2020.
18. Hall RCW. Exploitation of the elderly: undue influence as a form of elder abuse. Clin Geriatrics. 2005;13(2):28–35.
19. West's Encyclopedia of American Law online edition. Available from: http://www.encyclopedia.com/doc/1G2-3437704489.html.
20. Singer MT Undue influence and written documents: psychological aspects. Journal of Questioned Examination. 1992. Available from: http://www.csj.org/pub_csj/csj_vol10_no1_93/influence_written.htm. Accessed May 31 2020.
21. Testimony of Mickey Rooney, Senate Special Committee on Aging. March 2, 2011. Available from: https://www.aging.senate.gov/imo/media/doc/hr230mr.pdf.
22. Spar JE, Garb AS. Assessing competency to make a will. Am J Psychiatry. 1992;149:169–74.
23. Fulmer T, Guadagno L, Bitando-Dyer C, Connolly MT. Progress in elder abuse screening and assessment instruments. J Am Geriatr Soc. 2004;52:297–304.
24. Investor Protection Trust. Pocket guide on elder investment fraud and financial exploitation. Available from https://www.nasaa.org/wp-content/uploads/2011/08/EIFFE-Clinicians-Pocket-Guide.pdf. Accessed May 30 2020.

Chapter 3
Barriers to Recognition

Ronan M. Factora

> My money was stolen from me. I was eventually stripped of the ability to make even the most basic decisions… my daily life became unbearable [1].

Hollywood movie star Mickey Rooney's experience of being financially exploited was brought to the public eye during the Senate Special Committee on Aging, March 2, 2011. In spectacular fashion, he provided the grim details of how he was isolated and taken advantage financially of by none other than his family. Though his experience is not necessarily unique, the public attention to his testimony once again brought to light how vulnerable our older citizens are to this type of abuse.

Who Reports

Despite the studies of the prevalence and incidence of this problem (detailed in Chap. 1), the onus falls on the victim and those interacting with this individual to bring attention to the abuse.

Self-report of elder mistreatment of abuse, though, seldom occurs. Several studies find that 70% or more of cases of elder abuse are not self-reported. The responsibility thus falls on the community and those interacting with victims to report the abuse.

R. M. Factora (✉)
Cleveland Clinic Lerner College of Medicine at Case Western Reserve University, Cleveland Clinic, Cleveland, OH, USA
e-mail: factorr@ccf.org

R. M. Factora (ed.), *Aging and Money*,
https://doi.org/10.1007/978-3-030-67565-3_3

In all 50 states and the District of Columbia, mandatory reporting laws exist requiring those in the healthcare field to report *suspected or confirmed* elder abuse. Approximately 30 states require reporting only by persons specifically listed in that state's statute. The most common listed mandatory reporters include health care providers, human services providers, and law enforcement. Sixteen states require reporting by any person having reason to believe abuse has taken place. At least 30 states have penalties for failing to report elder abuse. This may include reporting a licensed professional's failure to maintain this obligation to the appropriate licensing board.

The definition of who is considered a mandated reporter varies from state to state, but can include more than just health care personnel and those involved in law enforcement. Table 3.1 lists the mandated reporters for the states of Ohio and California. Clearly, other disciplines beyond those involved in direct health care delivery may be obligated to report suspected abuse. This includes clergy, employees at adult day care facilities (which could include custodial staff, cafeteria staff), and (in California) employees of animal control services. Though not explicitly identified in California, individuals involved in the management of an elder's financial affairs (including those in the finance or banking industry) could fall into the category of "administrators, supervisors, and any licensed staff of a public or private facility that provides care or services for older persons or dependent adults." The addition of similar disciplines to the list of mandated reporters was implemented into the Ohio statues in 2019. It is important to be familiar with what the laws state in one's own residence.

When reported in good faith, mandated reporters are protected from litigation for reporting suspected abuse by state laws. Confidentiality of the mandated reporter is maintained to encourage greater reporting of suspected cases.

In one study looking at who reports suspected elder abuse, the vast majority of reports come from the community (Fig. 3.1). Social workers and mental health personnel comprise another large fraction of reporters, followed by non-physician health care workers. In this survey, physicians were the least likely to report any cases of abuse [2].

Table 3.1 Mandated reporters for suspected elder abuse (examples from Ohio and California)

Ohio: Any attorney, physician, osteopath, podiatrist, chiropractor, dentist, psychologist, hospital employee, licensed nurse, ambulatory health facility employee, home health agency employee, adult care facility employee, nursing home employee, residential care facility employee, home for the aging employee, senior service provider, peace officer, coroner, clergyman, community mental health facility employee, and a person engaged in social work or counseling. In 2019, the following professions were also added to the list of mandated reporters:
Pharmacists
Employees of outpatient health facilities
Firefighters
Employees of the health department
Ambulance drivers
First responders
Building inspectors

Table 3.1 (continued)

Certified public accountants
Bank, savings and loan, and credit union employees
Real estate brokers or agents
Notary publics
Investment advisors
Accredited financial planners
California: "Any person who has assumed full or intermittent responsibility for care or custody of an elder or dependent adult, whether or not that person receives compensation, including administrators, supervisors, and any licensed staff of a public or private facility that provides care or services for elder or dependent adults, or any elder or dependent adult care custodian, health practitioner, or employee of a county adult protective services agency or local law enforcement agency is a mandated reporter" (Welfare and Institutions Code Section 15630, see Appendix 5).
Examples of who must report:
Care custodians
Health practitioners
County welfare departments
Employees of law enforcement agencies
Employees of fire departments
Employees of humane societies and animal control agencies
Employees of environmental health and building code enforcement
Clergy members
Any other protective, public, sectarian, mental health, private assistance, or advocacy agency, or person providing health services or social services to elders or dependent adults
Any person who has assumed full or intermittent responsibility for care or custody of an elder or dependent adult

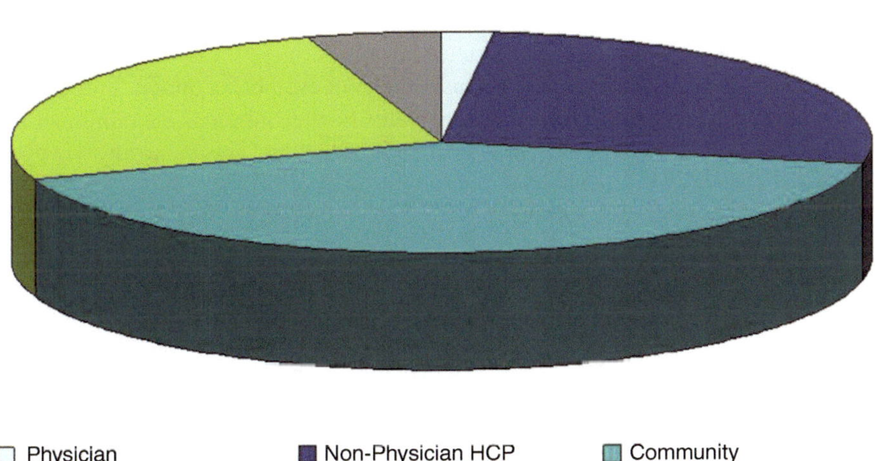

Fig. 3.1 Result of survey determining reporters for suspected elder abuse [2]

Barriers to Self-Reporting

Many reasons exist explaining why victims of elder abuse do not report the events.

Isolation of potential victims is often a barrier to detection and reporting of abuse. Abusers may achieve this by denying these persons physical access to friends, communication to friends and family (e.g. telephone, social media), or denying/preventing excursions from home except for medical visits. Contact with individuals outside of the home may be prohibited by the perpetrator through threatening behavior or by creating an environment of conflict that could make the visitors feel uncomfortable. Friends and family members who would be able to intervene may be driven away by this behavior, leaving the victim even more isolated. The perpetrator's behavior may subsequently escalate, leading to a perpetual cycle of isolation and abuse. One study comparing elder abuse victims with a control group found that abused older persons did appear more isolated [3], and they tended to have fewer overall contacts and to feel negatively about their social situations.

Victims of elder abuse may believe that they are responsible for the abuse or that they pose a burden on their caregivers. These feelings of lack of self-esteem represent this population's own "ageism" or feelings of self-blame. They may consequently feel that their mistreatment is deserved.

When a family member is the abuser, the victim often does not want to report them. These individuals often feel shame, guilt, and fear in these circumstances [4]. Some older persons may believe that occurrence of the abuse itself may be an indicator that they are no longer able to manage themselves independently, and that this may lead to the appointment of a guardian and further loss of independence. Domestic violence victims as well as elder abuse victims may be reluctant to change their situations, particularly for fear of ending up alone or putting the abuser at risk (e.g. incarcerated, homeless) as a result of filing a report. Many fear that institutionalization may be the only alternative solution to tolerating abuse, as the perpetrator may be the only individual that the victim may rely on.

As such, legal action against the abuser may not even be an option for the victim. Victims may demonstrate tremendous loyalty to their abuser and minimize their feelings and symptoms, even to their healthcare provider. This behavior may persist even if the issue is acknowledged or brought up at all by the victim. The value of these close personal ties often overrides any injury they may suffer from their perpetrators.

Cultural and language barriers may also prevent victims from reporting elder abuse and mistreatment. If individuals are not able to effectively describe or explain their circumstances to those they wish to report the abuse to, action may be limited. Lack of ability to speak English along with a fear of abandonment from their society may prevent reporting.

Various cultural groups traditionally hold elders in positions of respect and esteem. Often, elders expect to be cared for by family. When these members are no longer willing or able, the elders may become vulnerable to abuse. These obligations may even be resented by family members, leading to abusive situations [5]. Embarrassment on the part of the victim may prevent them from reporting abuse to a representative of their own community, much less individuals who are not of their cultural background. It is not uncommon for various cultural groups to feel that "outsiders should not be aware of their affairs," characterizing social welfare institutions as "alien," and making it more difficult for practitioners to detect any problems [6]

Observations of behavioral changes in an individual may provide clues regarding their risk and ability to make decisions [7]. Persons working with immigrants should be familiar with risk factors for elder abuse in these cultures so as to recognize them more readily and intervene when necessary. Cultural sensitivity is important in framing the suspected abuse in a fashion that is appropriate to individuals in different cultures and ethnic backgrounds. Utilization of interpreters or practitioners knowledgeable in the individual's language and culture may aide in providing services to these persons.

In some circumstances, cognitive impairment prevents victims from recognizing that the abuse is occurring. In other circumstances, such individuals may recognize what is going on but may not know how to go about reporting the events. Physical impairments or dependence upon the perpetrator to perform activities of daily living may also be a barrier to reporting. Often, patients themselves will choose to return to environments deemed unsafe. In these situations, staff members struggle to determine whether victims are exercising poor judgment or have crossed over the fine line to decisional incapacity. Determining whether individuals have the capacity to make appropriate decisions about remaining in these abusive situations is a challenge to practicing clinicians (See Chap. 7).

Barriers to Reporting

Physicians are in the front lines of patient care. They are the professionals in an ideal position to recognize and identify elder abuse and initiate a plan of care and communication with community services to manage suspected elder abuse. Despite this opportunity, surveys have often identified physicians as the individuals in health care least likely to report suspected elder abuse. Non-physician health care practitioners, social workers, and workers in the mental health field are much more likely to report than physicians [2]. Despite this wide array of persons mandated to report and intervene, common barriers to reporting are encountered by many disciplines.

A review of the literature identifying barriers preventing physicians from reporting elder abuse serves to highlight what persons in other disciplines may also encounter. In one survey of physicians conducted to determine why physicians did not report [8], the following barriers were acknowledged by the respondents:

- Abuse involved subtle signs: 44%
- Victim denied that abuse was going on: 23%
- Physician was unsure of reporting procedures: 21%
- Physician was unclear about reporting laws, definitions, accessing community resources: 10%

Physicians are trained to be aware of the prevalence of illnesses in the general population, so as to recognize them in clinical practice and initiate appropriate management. Though medical student training in pediatric medicine often involves training in the recognition of the signs of child abuse, few physicians have been trained to recognize signs of elder abuse [9, 10]. Distinguishing between aging and findings that are consistent with elder abuse (such as bruising patterns, weight loss, fractures) is important to support a clinician's clinical suspicion that abuse is occurring. Though the American Medical Association recommends screening for abuse in all elders [11], lack of training leads to clinicians who are unaware of the prevalence or abuse or the importance of screening for it in at-risk populations [12].

Lack of awareness of risk factors is compounded by a lack of appropriate documentation when elder abuse is recognized or occurring. Such documentation would be invaluable to investigators looking into suspected cases. The value of accurate documentation is dependent completely on the clinician's ability to recognize and document clinically significant findings and suspicions (See Chap. 10).

Physicians are often reluctant to ask about elder abuse; approach of this topic has been seen as akin to "opening Pandora's box" [13]. Busy practitioners are very sensitive to time constraints. A lack of time may prevent implementation of screening for elder abuse or providing patients with the opportunity to report it. Mandated reporters in various areas where at-risk individuals spend their time have significant difficulty recognizing abuse. Limited availability of brief and effective screening tools for elder abuse and knowledge of reporting procedures are also reported barriers, though developments in this area are advancing (See Chap. 8). When concerns are raised regarding the victim's ability to make appropriate decisions regarding their own safety, persons encountering this situation may not be familiar with how to conduct this evaluation (See Chap. 7).

Once abuse is identified, many may feel powerless to "fix" the problem. Mandated reporters may have the perception that government agencies will be unwilling or unable to help. They may be unaware of the existence of laws regarding elder abuse, including a lack of awareness that financial exploitation could be prosecuted as a criminal offense. Though removal of individuals from abusive situations may be possible, admission to the hospital for a "social admission" is difficult in the absence of another reimbursable reason for hospitalization.

For suspected victims of elder abuse who are in safe clinical settings like hospitals, another concern is the potential of sending the victim back to the environment where the abuse was taking place after discharge. Safety concerns for the at-risk person necessitate generating a plan of support upon return to the community. That person should also be given easy means of contacting emergency assistance if necessary. This plan requires knowledge on the part of the practitioner on what services are available and whom should be contacted, with the purpose of protecting the potential victim from any retaliation by the perpetrator (see Chap. 11). Offering medical home care services (when applicable) or connecting these individuals to additional community agencies that can support that individual at home may reduce the isolation that these individuals feel and provide opportunities by these agencies to report suspected abuse (to further protect these individuals).

Mandated reporters may also feel frightened or threatened by the abuser. Safety concerns may hinder involvement in abuse cases. Involvement of law enforcement in these circumstances may help reduce the potential for harm.

Eliminating Barriers

The barriers preventing recognition of elder abuse persist. There is a significant overlap in underlying causes of the barriers identified in victims as well as in mandated reporters. The range of causes, from lack of education on risk factors, lack of knowledge of reporting procedures and laws, and a lack of motivation to report, all contribute to the difficulty in recognizing and pursuing elder abuse in the community.

Education of the general public, clinicians, allied heath personnel, and any other individuals who are in direct contact and interact with vulnerable older persons (including clergy and those providing financial services to at-risk persons) is necessary to foster a greater recognition not just of the problem of elder abuse. Educating these persons also empowers them to be active in recognizing, reporting, and preventing abuse. Though many champions exist in these disciplines, funding priorities have often been cited as the underlying reason for a lack of resources to forward this agenda of advocacy. Beyond recognition, studies showing the efficacy of screening, interventions, and interaction between multidisciplinary and interdisciplinary teams tasked to investigate and manage elder abuse are greatly needed to bring more resources to prosecution of cases of elder abuse and prevention strategies to prevent abuse in those at risk.

Clearly, much work remains to bring the problem of elder abuse. Advocacy is the best way to bring more light to its victims (See Chap. 13).

References

1. Rooney M. Testimony of Mickey Rooney – senate special subcommittee on aging. Accessed at http://www.scnursinghomelaw.com/uploads/file/Mickey%20Rooney.pdf South Carolina Nursing Home Blog http://www.scnursinghomelaw.com/2011/03/articles/advocacy/justice-for-all-ending-elder-abuse-neglect-and-financial-exploitation/. March 2 2011.
2. Rosenblatt DE, Cho KH, Durance PW. Reporting mistreatment of older adults: the role of physicians. J Am Geriatr Soc. 1996;44(1):65–70.
3. Wolf RS, Pillemer K. Understanding the causes of physical elder abuse. In: Helping elderly victims: the reality of elder abuse. New York: Columbia University Press; 1989. p. 69–81.
4. Cammer Paris BE. Violence against elderly people. Mt Sinai J Med. 1996;63(2):97–100.
5. Montoya V. Understanding and combating elder abuse in Hispanic communities. J Elder Abuse Negl. 1997;9(2):5–17.

6. Brownell P. The application of the Culturagram in cross-cultural practice with elder abuse victims. J Elder Abuse Negl. 1997;9(2):19–33.
7. Baladerian NJ. Recognizing abuse and neglect in people with severe cognitive and/or communication impairments. J Elder Abuse Negl. 1997;9(2):93–104.
8. Kennedy RD. Elder abuse and neglect: the experience, knowledge, and attitudes of primary care physicians. Fam Med. 2005;37(7):481–5.
9. Warshaw C. Identification, assessment and intervention with victims of domestic violence. In: Warshaw C, Ganley AL, editors. Improving the health care response to domestic violence. A resource manual for health care providers. San Francisco; 1998. p. 49–86.
10. Alpert EJ, Tonkin AE, Seeherman AM, Holtz HA. Family violence curricula in US medical schools. Am J Prev Med. 1998;14(4):273–82.
11. American Medical Association. REPORT 7 OF THE COUNCIL ON SCIENCE AND PUBLIC HEALTH (A-08) elder mistreatment (resolution 429, A-07) (reference committee D). 2008.
12. Gerbert B, Caspers N, Bronstone A, Moe J, Abercrombie P. A qualitative analysis of how physicians with expertise in domestic violence approach the identification of victims. Ann Intern Med. 1999;131(8):578–84.
13. Sugg NK, Inui T. Primary care physicians' response to domestic violence. Opening Pandora's box. JAMA. 1992;267(23):3157–60.

Chapter 4
Risk Factors for Patient and Caregiver

Anthony Casacchia and Natalie Kayani

Ms. Jones was an 82-year-old frail woman with moderately severe-staged Alzheimer's dementia. She had been living alone in the community until her niece, Jane, moved in to assist with caregiving. Jane sought assistance from the Area Agency on Aging (AAoA) and a Geriatric Assessment Center to determine her aunt's needs, as well as community options for care giving. Ms. Jones was never married and had no assistance prior to Jane's involvement. Aside from Jane, no one else was listed on her contact forms with various hospitals and agencies. During the assessment, Ms. Jones did not remember her doctor's name or names of neighbors or friends. Referral to home health agencies was refused by Jane, who felt she could adequately provide for the patient's needs. Once Jane moved in, she took control of finances, using the car and money for her own needs, as well as the needs of Ms. Jones. Over the next few months, as Ms. Jones became more dependent, disabled, and cognitively impaired, Jane continued to refuse outside support. Despite obvious caregiver stress and lack of 24-hour care, no progress was made to convince Jane to increase her support system.

At the time of Ms. Jones' death, it was revealed that Jane was sole heir of the estate, valued at $750,000. It was also determined that Ms. Jones' Power of Attorney and Will had been written at a time when she lacked the decisional capacity for completing such documents. Neighbors relayed that Jane moved out during her final months. Ms. Jones was left alone without supervision and assistance. Neighbors worked together to provide around-the-clock care until her death.

Older adults visit health providers for medical or physical issues. An unstated concern during these visits might be financial exploitation. This can be challenging to determine. Abuse is often overlooked due to the providers' inability to recognize risk factors. Education on these risks and the importance of maintaining a high level of suspicion in order to recognize them are the first steps.

A. Casacchia · N. Kayani (✉)
Division of Geriatric Medicine, Summa Health System, Akron, OH, USA
e-mail: casacchiaa@summahealth.org; kayanin@summahealth.org

R. M. Factora (ed.), *Aging and Money*,
https://doi.org/10.1007/978-3-030-67565-3_4

There is consensus in published literature describing the "typical" victim of financial exploitation. Similar to other sources, the National Elder Abuse Center describes the typical victim as "between the ages of 70 and 89, white, female, frail, and cognitively impaired" [1]. This chapter reviews the literature on the risk factors for financial abuse of the elderly. Although there are limitations to the research, most studies reach the same conclusions about characteristics of the victim, perpetrators, and environment. Recognizing these potential red flags is an important step to limiting the abuse. We propose that the most effective approach involves using the expertise of an interdisciplinary team to uncover and recognize financial abuse. These team members can include physicians, nurse, social worker, pharmacist adult protective services, law enforcement, and attorneys. For the purpose of this chapter, we will focus on the medical model team–based approach to financial abuse of the elderly.

Risk Factor Recognition

Several risk factors associated with vulnerability to financial abuse have been identified, though published research addressing this issue has its limitations. Most studies are retrospective. Many of the larger studies were completed in the 1990s. Despite these drawbacks, several evidence-based factors are identified as placing older adults in jeopardy from financial abuse and show that the interplay of these risks (Fig. 4.1) may increase the vulnerability of an older person. Vulnerability is defined as "capable of or susceptible to being hurt" [2]. Although financial abuse can occur against those who are not vulnerable, proactively identifying those at highest risk may lead to actions to establish safeguards of protection. This requires ongoing education of professionals who may be the only outside contact for these individuals.

Victim's Risk Factors

Age: Ms. Jones Is an 82-Year-Old Frail Woman…

A large study on elder abuse of all types concluded that advanced age is linked to an increased likelihood for financial abuse [3]. In one study, 48% of the victims were 80 years or older, followed by 28.7% aged 75–79 years old, 10.8% aged 70–74 years old, and 9.4% aged 65–69 years. Additionally, the oldest group of 80 years and above constituted a quarter of all types of elder abuse victims. At the time of this study's publication in 1996, this population comprised only 19% of the total elderly in the country. A more recent study in 2009 by Garre-Olmo et al. analyzed the

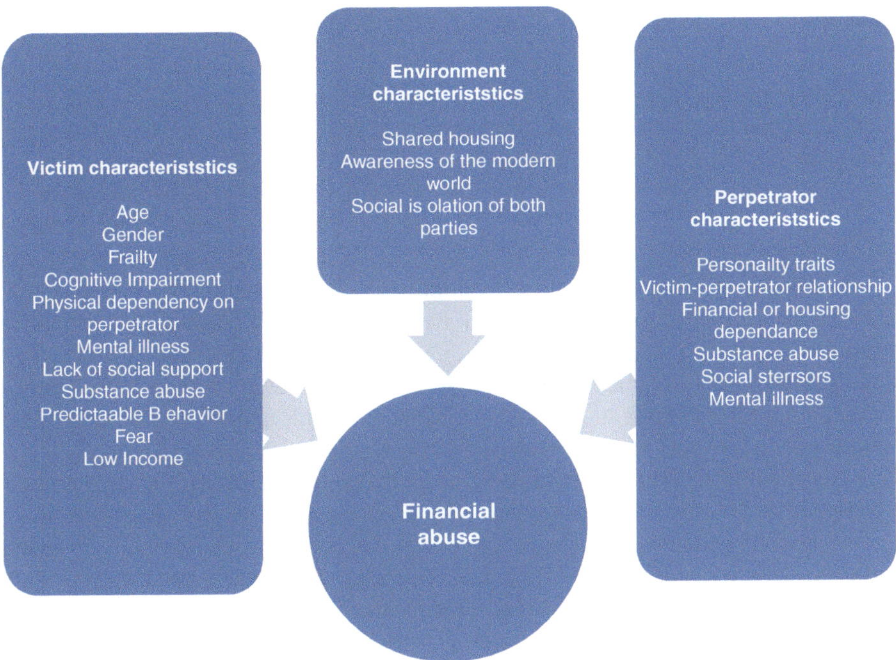

Fig. 4.1 Relationship between victim, perpetrator, and environmental factors in elder abuse

prevalence and risk factors for financial abuse in a population in rural Spain [4]. In this study, those aged 85 or older had a higher risk of financial abuse compared to those under 85 years old, with the study demonstrating an odds ratio (OR) of 3.84 (95% CI 1.70–8.68) supporting this observation.

Other recent studies show that more advanced age may not be as strongly linked. A study by Laumann et al. in 2008 (based on the National Social Life, Health and Aging Project) found that 3.5% of 3005 surveyed older adults reported financial mistreatment [5]. Analysis of this cohort showed a negative association of age with the odds of reporting financial mistreatment (OR 0.95, $p < 0.05$). Another study by Acierno et al. in 2010 (based on the National Elder Mistreatment Study which included the interview responses of 5777 older adults) found that respondents aged <70 years were more likely reported to having fallen victim to financial mistreatment by strangers [6].

Possible explanations for these discordant findings include methodologies of data collection and cultural differences. In the 1996 study, prevalence data was gathered from Adult Protective Services records and sentinel reports [3]. In the conflicting studies in 2008 and 2010, adults were methodically sampled and data gathered by direct interviews or surveys, representing direct patient reports of mistreatment [5, 6]. Differences in recall, perceptions of personal experiences, or definitions of financial mistreatment may contribute to these findings.

Gender: Ms. Jones Is an 82-Year-Old Frail Woman…

In 1996, women comprised 57.6% of the US population aged 60 and older. However, the proportion of female financial abuse victims totaled 63% [3]. In contrast, the National Elderly Abuse Incident Study (NEAIS) in 1998 showed that the greatest gender disparity was in the area of financial abuse where 92% of its victims were women. The proportion of female abuse victims identified in this study is striking.

Internationally, this trend generally continues. A review article by Pillemer et al. also found women to have a higher risk for financial exploitation in multiple international studies [7]. However, a study in a population in Korea showed men more likely to be victims of financial exploitation [7], and a large study in Japan showed women with lower odds of experiencing financial exploitation [8]. Cultural differences may contribute to these discordant findings.

The reason why women are often disproportionately victims of financial abuse is complicated. Historically, society has viewed women as "weaker" and "less financially astute" than men. This perception was likely due to the division of gender roles in which men typically handled the finances. The identification of women in this way identifies them as easy targets for financial abuse by predators.

Race and Ethnicity

Several studies have shown disparities in the prevalence of financial exploitation when comparing different racial and ethnic groups. Several studies show an increased risk of financial exploitation of African Americans compared to Caucasians [5, 7, 9, 10]. In a 2014 prevalence study based in New York State, African Americans experienced financial exploitation more frequently compared to Caucasians in 1 year period, with this study demonstrating a relative risk (RR) of 3.80 (95% CI 1.11–13.04) for financial exploitation within 1 year. It also estimated a lifetime RR of 2.61 (95% CI 0.84–4.70) for financial exploitation in African Americans compared to Caucasians [9]. A 2008 study by Laumann et al. (based on the National Social Life, Health and Aging Project where 3005 respondents were interviewed) found greater odds that African Americans would experience financial exploitation compared to Caucasians (OR 1.77, $p < 0.05$) [5].

In contrast, Latino ethnicity is associated with decreased prevalence of financial exploitation [5, 7]. In the same 2008 study by Laumann et al., Latino ethnicity was associated with an OR of 0.22 ($p < 0.05$) of financial exploitation when compared to Caucasians [5].

Frailty: ...as Ms. Jones Became More Dependent...

Anecdotal and clinical reports have suggested that frailty contributes to an older individual's vulnerability to abuse. Financial abuse in frail older persons has not been assessed in any longitudinal studies [11–13]. Frailty may hinder a victim's ability to report the financial exploitation. Additionally, it is reasonable to assume the predator believes the victim will not live long enough to report the abuse [14, 15]. Red flags of vulnerability include the use of handicapped placards, canes, walkers, and other assistive devices.

Cognitive Impairment: ...as Ms. Jones Became More... Cognitively Impaired...

Dementia increases with age, which might affect one's ability to manage finances. Cognitive impairment has been identified as a risk factor for abuse due to its effect on decision-making capacity, judgment, and memory [16]. Individuals with poor reasoning ability and memory impairment are more susceptible to a variety of influences [17]. Numeracy and numerical reasoning can decline with age and contribute to worse decision-making regarding finances [18]. In a study by Wood et al. in 2016, higher numeracy, assessed by an 11-item scale focused on numerical literacy, was associated with decreased risk of financial exploitation after controlling for other demographic variables [19]. Fraud victims have an increased risk of a diagnosis of dementia and poor executive and calculation function. In general, higher cognitive abilities allow planning for the future and participation in finances [18]. Consistent with this, dementia-associated cognitive decline is a significant risk factor for both financial abuse and the reporting of abuse [4, 16, 20, 21].

Physical Dependency: ....as Ms. Jones Became More ...Disabled

Research has shown that dependency increases the incidence of all types of abuse [22]. The NEAIS report suggested that a large proportion (about three out of four) of elder abuse and neglect victims suffer from physical frailty [3]. Need for ADL assistance has been associated with financial mistreatment by family [6, 10]. The presence of physical disabilities, such as severe limitations with basic and/or instrumental activities of daily living, or significant sensory impairment creates dependency on others. As an example, physically dependent adults typically rely on others to assist with financial transactions, such as bill paying or cashing checks. Overall, health and functional status presents complex risk factors for financial abuse and are difficult to evaluate individually.

Mental Illness

Published medical literature has demonstrated a strong link between mental illness and an increased risk for abuse. Such research indicates that older adults with advanced mental or psychiatric illness have increased chances of dependency and abuse [20, 23–25]. Mental illness decreases the capacity to recognize the abuse and the ability to report it. The effects of financial abuse on the mentally ill, who are more likely to be poor, can be particularly devastating [26–29]. In addition, the distress of abuse can exacerbate symptoms and lead to increased isolation and social exclusion [28, 30, 31]. Specifically, depression is a significant predictor of elder financial abuse [8, 32–34]. According to the National Alliance on Mental Illness, 19% of older Americans are affected by depression [35]. Mental illness in the older adult is a potential red flag for abuse.

Lack of Social Support: …She Had Been Living Alone…

Having few social contacts is a risk factor for abuse of older persons. Acierno et al. [6] reported in the National Elder Mistreatment Study that all types of abuse correlate with low social support. Specifically, the report stated "Low social support was associated with more than triple the likelihood that mistreatment of any form would be reported" [6 , p.295]. A study by Phillips [13] also found that abused older adults are more socially isolated [13]. A 2017 study by Liu et al. with 395 community-dwelling older adults found negative interactions with close social network members, and lower perceived social support were associated with a higher risk of financial exploitation [36]. In addition to its identity as a risk factor, low social support is linked to concealment of abuse. In contrast, Bonnie and Wallace [37] hypothesized that such illicit behaviors are less likely to occur in strong connected families [37].

Quinn (1997) suggests that the best method to deter undue influence is encouraging social interactions [38]. Being active in community affairs, participating in volunteering activities, and attending senior centers or church can contribute to an active social life. Similarly, having many friends and trusted acquaintances increases the odds that unusual activity will be noted. As examples, a long-time banker notices changes in banking patterns, or close friends become suspicious of strangers who are quickly involved in an older adult's personal affairs. In conclusion, it is important for providers to recognize the social milieu of older adults.

Substance Abuse

Substance abuse has been implicated as the most common predisposing factor in all types of elder abuse [39, 40]. However, association of a victim's substance abuse to that same individual experiencing financial exploitation specifically is less clear. In a 1996 study by Hwalek et al., it was found that victim substance abuse was associated with perpetrator substance abuse [41]. This may lead to increased financial abuse as perpetrator substance use is a known risk factor. In contrast, Tredal et al. found in 2012 that victim alcohol abuse was associated with a lower risk of financial abuse in a European cohort [42]. Finally, a 2016 cross-sectional study by Conrad et al. found that although perpetrator substance abuse was associated with increased financial exploitation, victim substance abuse did not affect the risk of financial abuse [43]. This study also did not support the finding of an association of perpetrator and victim substance abuse rates. Further study of this issue is indicated.

Fear

Mr. Smith, a 79–year-old man with Alzheimer's, was admitted to the hospital due to an exacerbation of asthma. Six months prior to this hospitalization, an elderly woman with dementia and her daughter, Kelly, moved in with Mr. Smith. Kelly assumed caregiving roles for Mr. Smith and her mother. Mr. Smith's son, who lived out of state, paid Kelly to provide care for his dad. After two subsequent hospitalizations for failure to thrive, a referral was made to Adult Protective Services. The investigator found poor living conditions and inadequate provisions for basic needs. They uncovered that Mr. Smith did not report this abuse and was fearful of the alternative options for care. He knew that not having Kelly meant he would need a nursing home.

Fear, in its numerous forms, can dissuade a victim from reporting abuse. These manifestations include the following: fear of being abandoned, retaliation from the perpetrator, fear of not being believed, fear of getting a loved one into trouble, fear of being stigmatized as victim, fear of being deemed incompetent [25, 44].

The experience of loneliness of an elderly victim and a desire for companionship increase the susceptibility to perpetrators [25]. The victim may be reluctant to report abuse because of the perceived value of the relationship to the perpetrator and embarrassment at being scammed and appearing gullible [28]. Another deterrent to reporting is the fear of being found incapable of managing finances and being placed in a nursing home [25].

Fear of change in residence can influence a victim's willingness to report abuse. Some victims might prefer to continue to remain in an abusive situation so they can remain in their current living situation [45]. Many victims assume abuse is a one-time event and may not realize it can be a pattern of repeated behavior [16, 29, 46].

Family ties can be a barrier to reporting as well. It is often difficult for a victim to report abuse when a family member is the perpetrator [14, 25]. In summary, fear of isolation and loyalty to the relationship increase the risk for abuse.

Low Income

Income is not a risk factor in the sense one would expect. Older adults with higher incomes are not at an increased risk for exploitation. However, having a low income is a risk factor [7, 9]. The National Elder Abuse Incident Study reported that about half of the victims of financial abuse had low incomes between $5000 and $14,000 [3].

Perpetrator Characteristics

A review of the literature suggests that perpetrators include a wide range of individuals. These include family members, friends, neighbors, caregivers, and strangers. A study by Tueth [23] describes two perpetrator types. The first type's characteristics include low self-esteem, mental health issues, and/or substance abuse problems. They may also be suffering from caregiver stress. These individuals do not actively seek the victims [23]. The second type of perpetrator is described as more aggressive. Individuals falling into this "type" utilize tactics of isolation, power, and control over the victim. Abuse is accomplished employing methods of intimidation, deceit, and other forms of psychological abuse [23]. In a 2006 article by Kemp and Liao, three types of perpetrator abuse are described. These include the opportunist, the family member, and the professional scam artist [47]. The opportunist can include paid caregivers, accountants, contractors, clergy, neighbors, stockbrokers, and attorneys who discover a person they can take advantage of. Family members that become perpetrators typically come from a history of family discord. Official scam artists make a living off of taking advantage of older people.

Understanding the characteristics of perpetrators, regardless of their relationship to the victim, could be helpful in identification. Unfortunately, scant research exists that profiles perpetrator characteristics. Field professionals have generated a list of possible factors based on speculations. Rabiner et al. [48] identified a set of four factors commonly associated with all forms of abuse by the perpetrator [48]. These include substance abuse, mental health issues, gambling behavior, and financial problems. This section explores perpetrator characteristics such as personality traits, victim-perpetrator relationship, financial or housing dependence, social stressors such as isolation, unemployment, divorce, and unstable relationships [48].

Personality of the Abuser

Hall et al. [49] provided profiles for male and female perpetrators of financial abuse. The male profile includes the personality traits of sociopathic and dependent [27]. The profile for the female predator includes the following traits: protector, opportunistic, predatory, and antisocial [49]. In addition, most literature identified perpetrators as a single male, younger than the victim, with a sense of entitlement [49]. This feeling of entitlement leads some perpetrators to believe that they will eventually inherit the assets and see this as justification for the abuse [45]. Others believe that they are getting paid for the care and services they are providing to the older adult [45].

Victim Perpetrator Relationship

Financial abuse is predominantly perpetrated by family members, especially adult children and caregivers. In 30% of cases, the perpetrator of financial abuse is a family member or a close relative of the victim [33, 48]. Of the cases that were reported to Adult Protective Services (APS), 60% were perpetrated by adult children [1]. Another prevalence study based in New York State based on 4156 adults published in 2014 showed that 57.9% of perpetrators were family members, with adult children making up 24.6% of the perpetrators in these cases [9]. Studies also reported that the likelihood of financial abuse by an adult male child is 2.5 times higher than the same type of abuse by a female child [33].

On the other hand, strangers might exploit without any close contact with the victim [50]. Examples include telemarketing and bank fraud, home repair scams, and borrowing money. When evaluating a potential victim of older abuse, it should be kept in mind that although victims of telemarketing and internet scams get the most media attention, it is often family and friends that are the most frequent perpetrators of such abuse (Table 4.1).

Financial Dependence

Published literature reports that an increased likelihood of financial exploitation is associated with the financial dependence of the perpetrator on the victim [7, 51–54]. One community agency survey of elder abuse cases in Massachusetts identified a "web of mutual dependency" between abuser and abused [51]. In two-thirds of the cases, the perpetrator was financially dependent on the victim. These findings were in agreement with other studies [55, 56]. During an assessment of a potential victim of financial abuse, it is important to uncover the extent of financial dependency between victim and suspected perpetrator. Financial interdependency should raise a red flag for the potential of abuse. Questions regarding older adults' resources and assets should be a standard part of the evaluation.

Table 4.1 Relationship of perpetrators to victims (based on one study of substantiated Adult Protective Services Cases)

Non-institutional perpetrators	
Family, Caregivers, and Friends (total 82)	
Family:	45
Son:	18
Daughter:	7
Nephew/Niece:	7
Granddaughter/Grandson:	6
Other relatives:	6
Fictive Kin:	1
(i.e., non-relatives considered to be "like" family)	
Caregiver (non-agency):	29
Neighbor/Friend:	8
Others (total 65)	
Befriended:	15 ("Sweetheart Scam")
Stranger:	14
Contractors:	12
Handyman/Chores/Caretaker:	9
Con Man:	5
Home Repair Scam:	4
Phone Scams:	4
"Travelers":	2
Criminal (total 8)	
Robber/Burglar:	4
Transient:	2
Serial Rapist:	1
Drugs:	1
Institutional Perpetrators	
Trusted Professionals (total 48)	
Financial:	33
Attorney/Paralegal:	11
Pastor/Minister:	2
Executors/Trustees:	1
CPA:	1
Other (total 63)	
Caregiver/Agency/Facility:	25
SNF/ALF/Personal Care Home Owner/Operator/Business Manager:	20
Medicare/Medicaid Fraud:	15
Health Care Fraud:	1
Hearing Aid Business:	1
Therapist:	1

Adapted from: Metlife. *Broken trust: elders, family and finances*. 2009.

Substance Abuse

A wealth of published research demonstrates a strong link between perpetrators and substance abuse. Several case-controlled and cross-sectional studies describe the disproportionate rate of substance abuse in older adult abuse perpetrators [7, 11, 43, 57, 58]. Additional studies of cases of elder abuse indicate that caregivers with substance abuse are involved in at least one-third of these cases [54, 59].

Social Stressors

Most of the perpetrators of financial abuse are identified as having social stressors. Life events such as unemployment, unstable relationships, or separation may increase the risk of a perpetrator committing an abuse against an older person. Some of the characteristics of such perpetrators include frequent switching of jobs, economic dependence on their victim, and isolation with minimal contact with the society [20].

Mental Illness

Depression among adult perpetrators of elderly victims has been identified as a risk factor [32]. A study published by Wolf and Pillemer [56] found that 40.7% of abusers had a history of mental illness [59]. In addition, a more recent study compared different types of abuse based on the data collected from APS agencies in Virginia. The results showed that 25% of the perpetrators had confirmed psychological diagnosis [60].

The Environment

It is vital to understand that abuse is not dependent on perpetrator and victim characteristics alone. Environmental factors also increase the risk for financial abuse. Living situations and attentiveness to surroundings as described below can increase risk.

Living Situation

Wolf and Pillemer discuss the risks of living situations in their book, *Helping Elderly Victims: The Reality of Elder Abuse*. They note that there is risk associated with living alone as well as living with others. Older persons who are living alone are more susceptible to victimization by strangers, whereas those living with families are most likely to be victimized by relatives, typically adult children. The authors reason that in a shared residence, the opportunities of contact (and consequently conflict) will be higher and increase the risk of mistreatment by those living in the same residence. Interestingly, they also note that the risk for financial abuse in living situations when an older person is alone is higher than for the other forms of elder abuse [56]. In a 2014 prevalence study in New York State, being an older adult living with a spouse was protective in a multivariate regression model for lifetime prevalence of financial exploitation (RR 0.39, 95% CI 0.26–0.59) [9].

Awareness of the Modern World

A lack of awareness of the modern world and modern financial practices may make an older person more vulnerable to financial exploitation [61]. Advances in modern technology, such as online banking, pose challenges for some older adults who are not familiar with their use. Complicated financial transactions such as reverse mortgages may also be more difficult for older individuals to understand, particularly if they are less financially savvy, have never managed financial affairs, or who have cognitive impairment that limits their understanding of the subject matter. Perpetrators may utilize these gaps in awareness or understanding present in an older person to take advantage of them.

Into Action: A Team-Based Approach

While the risk factors of the victim, perpetrator and environment involved in financial abuse of older adults appear broad and variable, an astute interdisciplinary team may recognize the patterns and characteristics present in the cases they encounter. Focused interviews from multiple disciplines uncover the biopsychosocial forces at play. Communication of risk factors in an educated team increases suspicion of financial abuse. Their job is to initiate an investigation and/or implement changes to reduce the risk.

The use of a team-based approach to risk recognition is recommended for effective care. Utilizing the unique skill sets of different professions (such as social work, nursing, medicine, adult protective services, and law enforcement) increases the probability that risks will be identified. Research results indicate that identification of elder abuse is improved through collaboration of professionals in a team setting. An example is found in Ernst [62]. The results of this study of elder maltreatment included increased risk reduction with the use of a team of a social worker and a nurse as compared to a social worker only [62]. Additional research supports the team approach for this issue. Dyer et al. [63] describes successful collaboration between members of a geriatric assessment team for the treatment of elder abuse. This team included geriatricians, geriatric nurse practitioners, social workers, and Adult Protective Service workers [63]. The dynamic of an interdisciplinary team combines individual areas of expertise, communication, and consensus regarding treatment plans. The case below illustrates how this works in risk recognition.

Mrs. Adams is an 83-year-old Caucasian woman with limited mobility due to spinal stenosis and chronic pain. She is brought in to the office for assessment of agitation, as reported by her son, Jim. The physician spends time with Jim and Mrs. Adams together and separately and concludes that Mrs. Adams has moderately severe dementia. It is recommended that she have supervision of medication administration, meal preparation, bathing, dressing, and financial management. Physical therapy is recommended to improve her mobility and decrease back pain.

Social work assessment of the situation reveals that Jim has always lived with his mother. He was never financially independent because of ongoing substance abuse problems. Over the years, he has provided progressively more support to his declining mother, causing an increase in his caregiver stress levels.

The pharmacist identifies medication that could be contributing to cognitive and physical decline and recommends alternative medications.

Nursing uncovers urinary incontinence and lack of awareness as a major stress on Jim. The nurse is able to convince Mrs. Adams to trial undergarment incontinence protection pads.

At the conclusion of the visit, the interdisciplinary team discusses their concerns. They recognize many risk factors for potential financial abuse. These include Mrs. Adams' age, gender, frailty, cognitive impairment, and physical dependency. In addition, the team considers Jim's stress, substance abuse, and financial dependency. The team's recommendations should improve Mrs. Adams physical dependency and reduces Jim's stress. The team will monitor the situation over time and watch for new flags of financial abuse.

At a follow-up visit, Jim reports reduction in stress as result of medication changes and incontinence management but remains stressed due to his mother's progressive dependence on him. Social work recommends applying for the Home Based Care Medicaid Waiver program to assist with Mrs. Adams needs, but Jim turns it down when he becomes aware of the Estate Recovery Program. This program would entitle the state to receive Mrs. Adams house at the time of Jim's death. Jim feels he is entitled to pass that asset to his heirs in exchange for the help he has provided his mother over the years.

Over the next few months, Mrs. Adams appeared increasingly unkempt and began to lose weight. Jim also appeared haggard yet declined any outside assistance. A referral was made to Adult Protective Services, who in turn applied for third-party guardianship of Mrs. Adams' person and estate. Jim's brother supported him through drug rehab and Mrs. Adams was moved to an Assisted Living (AL) facility by her guardian. With the sale of her house and a small savings, she was able to remain in AL until the time of her death 2 years later. Her son was able to get the help he needed with a previously undiagnosed mental health illness and live independently with the help of state assistance.

Conclusion

The identification of risk factors in suspected cases of elder abuse and financial exploitation is both complex and challenging. Risk factors for financial exploitation may be identifiable and recognizable in the potential victim, the perpetrator, and within the environment where the exploitation takes place. A team-based approach is the most effective way to identify these factors. Although the typical victim is a frail, older female with cognitive impairment and physical dependence, some that fit this profile legitimately exchange money for assistance, from family or strangers. The key to identifying those at risk of financial abuse is to recognize the pattern of victim, perpetrator, and environment and use the skills of the interdisciplinary team to intervene before the abuse has started. Continued education of professionals who can contribute to teams tackling this issue is needed to ensure that such cases are addressed appropriately when encountered.

References

1. National Center on Elder Abuse [NCEA]. The national elder abuse incidence study: final report. Washington, DC: National Aging Information Center; 1998.
2. Collins English Dictionary - Complete & Unabridged 10th Edition. Source location: HarperCollins Publishers. http://dictionary.reference.com/browse/vulnerability. Accessed 28 Dec 2019.
3. US Department of Health and Human Services Administration on Aging and the Administration for Children and Families. The national elder abuse incident study. Washington, DC: NCEA; 1998.
4. Garre-Olmo J, Planas-Pujol X, López-Pousa S, Juvinyà D, Vilà A, Vilalta-Franch J. Prevalence and risk factors of suspected elder abuse subtypes in people aged 75 and older. J Am Geriatr Soc. 2009;57:815–22.
5. Laumann EO, Leitsch SA, Waite LJ. Elder mistreatment in the United States: prevalence estimates from a nationally representative study. J Gerontol B Psychol Sci Soc Sci. 2008;63(4):S248–54.
6. Acierno R, Hernandez MA, Amstadter AB, Resnick HS, Steve K, Muzzy W, Kilpatrick DG. Prevalence and correlates of emotional, physical, sexual, and financial abuse and potential neglect in the United States: the National Elder Mistreatment Study. Am J Public Health. 2010;100(2):292–7.
7. Pillemer K, Burnes D, Riffin C, Lachs MS. Elder abuse: global situation, risk factors, and prevention strategies. Gerontologist. 2016;56(S2):S194–205.

8. Koga C, Hanazato M, Tsuji T, Suzuki N, Kondo K. Elder abuse and social capital in older adults: the Japan gerontological evaluation study. Gerontology. 2019;66:1–11.
9. Peterson JC, Burnes DPR, Caccamise PL, Mason A, Henderson CR, Wells MT, Berman J, Cook AM, Shukoff D, Brownell P, Powel M, Salamone A, Pillemer KA, Lachs MS. Financial exploitation of older adults: a population-based prevalence study. J Gen Intern Med. 2014;29(12):1615–23.
10. Acierno R, Hernandez-Tejada M, Muzzy W, Steve K. The final report: national elder mistreatment study. Washington, DC: US Department of Justice; 2009. Retrieved from: https://www.ncjrs.gov/pdffiles1/nij/grants/226456.pdf.
11. Bristowe E, Collins JB. Family-mediated abuse of non-institutionalized elder men and women living in British Columbia. J Elder Abuse Negl. 1989;1:45–54.
12. Paveza GJ, Cohen D, Eisdorfer C, Freels S, Semla T, Ashford W, et al. Severe family violence and Alzheimer's disease: prevalence and risk factors. Gerontologist. 1992;32(4):493–7.
13. Phillips LR. Elder abuse: what is it? Who says so? Geriatr Nurs. 1983;4:167–70.
14. Central California Legal Services [CCLS]. Elder financial abuse. 2001. Retrieved from: http://www.las.org/abuse/elderfinancial.html.
15. Chan TC, Luk JKH, Chiu PKC, Chan FHW, Chu LW. Financial abuse in a mentally incapacitated old man. Hong Kong Med J. 2009;15(3):213–6.
16. Wilber KH, Reynolds SL. Introducing a framework for defining financial abuse of the elderly. J Elder Abuse Negl. 1996;8:61–80.
17. Appelbaum PS, Grisso T. Assessing patients' capacities to consent to treatment. N Engl J Med. 1988;319(25):1635–8.
18. Wood S, Lichtenberg PA. Financial capacity and financial exploitation of older adults: research findings, policy recommendations, and clinical implications. Clin Gerontol. 2017;40(1):3–13.
19. Wood SA, Lui P, Hanoch Y, Estevez-Cores S. Importance of numeracy as a risk factor for elder financial exploitation in a community sample. J Gerontol B Psychol Sci Soc Sci. 2016;71(6):978–86.
20. Choi NG, Kulick DB, Mayer J. Financial exploitation of elders: analysis of risk factors based on county adult protective services data. J Elder Abuse Negl. 1999;10(3/4):39–62.
21. Podnieks E. National survey on abuse of the elderly in Canadian. J Elder Abuse Negl. 1992;4:5–58.
22. Lachs MS, Pillemer K. Current concepts : abuse and neglect of elderly persons. N Engl J Med. 1995;332(7):437–43.
23. Tueth MJ. Exposing financial exploitation of impaired elderly persons. Am J Geriatr Psychiatry. 2000;8(2):104–11.
24. Hafemeister T. Financial abuse of the elderly in domestic settings. In: Bonnie RL, Wallace RB, editors. Elder maltreatment: abuse, neglect, and exploitation in an aging America. Washington, DC: The National Academies Press; 2003. p. 382–445.
25. Hwang MM. Durable power of attorney: financial planning tool or license to steal? J Long Term Home Health Care. 1996;15:13–23.
26. Moskowitz S. New remedies for elder abuse and neglect. Probate Prop. 1998;12:52–6.
27. Smith RS. Fraud & financial abuse of older persons, 132. Canberra: Australian Institute of Criminology; 1999.
28. Coker J, Little B. Investing in the future: protecting the elderly from financial abuse. FBI Law Enforc Bull. 1997;66(12):1–5.
29. Nerenberg L. Developing a service response to elder abuse. Generations. 2000;24:86–92.
30. Deem DL. Notes from the field: observations in working with the forgotten victims of personal financial crimes. J Elder Abuse Negl. 2000;12(2):33–48.
31. Fielo SB. How does crime affect the elderly? Most crimes against the elderly are sustained by the inner-city aged who lives alone. Geriatr Nurs. 1987;1:80–3.
32. Beach SR, Shulz R, Castle NG, Rosen J. Financial exploitation and psychological mistreatment among older adults: differences between African Americans and non-African Americans in a population-based survey. Gerontologist. 2010;50(6):744–57.

33. MetLife Mature Market Institute, National Committee for the Prevention of Elder Abuse, & the Center for Gerontology at Virginia Polytechnic Institute and State University. Broken trust: elders, family, and finances. 2009. Retrieved from: https://www.giaging.org/documents/mmi-study-broken-trust-elders-family-finances.pdf.
34. MetLife. Elder financial abuse – crimes of occasion, desperation, and predation against America's elders; 2011.
35. National Alliance on Mental Illness. Depression in older persons fact sheet. Accessed 28 Dec 2019 from https://www.ncoa.org/resources/depression-in-older-persons-fact-sheet/.
36. Liu P, Wood S, Xi P, Berger DE, Wilber K. The role of social support in elder financial exploitation using a community sample. Innov Aging. 2017;100:1–11.
37. Bonnie RJ, Wallace RB, editors. Elder abuse: abuse, neglect and exploitation in an aging America. Washington, DC: National Academy Press; 2002.
38. Quinn MJ, Tomita SK. Elder abuse and neglect: causes, diagnosis and intervention strategies. 2nd ed. New York City: Springer; 1997.
39. World Health Organization. European report on preventing elder maltreatment. 2011. Available at http://www.euro.who.int/__data/assets/pdf_file/0010/144676/e95110.pdf.
40. Richardson B, Kitchen G, Livingstone G. The effect of education on knowledge and management of elder abuse: a randomized controlled trial. Age Ageing. 2002;31:335–41.
41. Hwalek MA, Neal AV, Goodrich C, Quinn K. The association of elder abuse and substance abuse in the Illinois elder abuse system. Gerontologist. 1996;36(5):694–700.
42. Tredal I, Soares JJF, Sundin Ö, Viitasara E, Melchiorre MG, Torres-Gonzales F, Stankunas M, Lindert J, Ioannidi-Kapolou E, Barros H. Alcohol use among abused and non-abused older persons aged 60–84 years: an European study. Drugs (Abingdon Engl). 2013;20(2):1–14.
43. Conrad KJ, Liu P, Iris M. Examining the role of substance abuse in elder mistreatment: results from mistreatment investigations. J Interpers Violence. 2016;34(2):1–26.
44. Shulman RW, Faierman-Shulman CA. Elder financial Abuse: a review for primary care physicians. Can Alzheimer Dis Rev. 2000;4:8–11.
45. Dessin CL. Financial abuse of the elderly. Idaho Law Rev. 2000;36:203–26.
46. National Clearinghouse on Family Violence [NCFV], Health Canada. Financial abuse of older adults. 2001. Retrieved from: http://publications.gc.ca/pub?id=9.572904&sl=0 9.572904&sl=0.
47. Kemp B, Liao S. Elder financial abuse: tips for the medical director. J Am Med Dir Assoc. 2006;7(9):591–3.
48. Rabiner D, O'Keefe J, Brown D. A conceptual framework of financial exploitation of older persons. J Elder Abuse Negl. 2005;16(2):53–73.
49. Hall RC, Hall RC, Chapman MJ. Exploitation of the elderly: undue influence as a form of elder abuse. Clin Geriatr. 2005;13(2):28–36.
50. US Administration on Aging. Financial exploitation of older persons: report to Congress; 2009.
51. Wolf R, Strugnell C, Godkin M. Preliminary findings from three model projects on elder abuse. Worcester: University Center on Aging, Massachusetts Medical Center; 1982.
52. Hwalek M, Hill B, Stahl C. Illinois plan for a statewide abuse program. In: Filinson R, Ingman S, editors. Elder abuse: practice and policy. New York: Human Services Press; 1989. p. 196–207.
53. Anetzberger GJ. Etiology of elder abuse by adult offspring. Springfield: Charles C. Thomas; 1987.
54. Greenberg JR, Mckibben M, Raymond JA. Dependent adult children and elder abuse. J Elder Abuse Negl. 1990;2(2):73–86.
55. Pillemer KA. Risk factors in elder abuse: results from a case-control study. In: Pillemer KA, Wolf RS, editors. Elder abuse: conflict in the family. Dover: Auburn House Publishing Company; 1986.
56. Wolf RS, Pillemer KA. Helping elderly victims: the reality of elder abuse. New York: Columbia University Press; 1989.

57. Lachs MS, et al. Risk factors for reported elder abuse and neglect: a nine-year observational cohort study. Gerontologist. 1997;37:469–74.
58. Wolfe DA, Zak L, Wilson S, Jaffe P. Child witnesses to violence between parents: critical issues in behavioral and social adjustment. J Abnorm Child Psychol. 1986;14(1):95–104.
59. Godkin MA, Wolf RS, Pillemer KA. A case-comparison analysis of elder abuse and neglect. Int J Aging Hum Dev. 1989;28:207–25.
60. Jackson S, Hafemeister T. Financial abuse of elderly people vs. other forms of elder abuse: assessing their dynamics, risk factors, and society's response. Final Report presented to the National Institute of Justice. August 2010. https://www.ncjrs.gov/pdffiles1/nij/grants/233613.pdf.
61. The Social Care Institute for Excellence. Assessment: financial crime against vulnerable adults. 2011. Available at www.scie.org.uk.
62. Ernst J, Smith CA. Assessment in adult protective services: do multidisciplinary teams made a difference? J Gerontol Soc Work. 2012;55(1):21–38.
63. Dyer CB, Gleason MS, Murphy KP, Pavlik VN, Portal B, Regev T, Hyman DJ. Treating elder neglect: collaboration between a geriatrics assessment team an adult protective services. South Med J. 1999;92(2):242–4.

Chapter 5
Aging and Financial Exploitation Risk

R. Nathan Spreng, Natalie C. Ebner, Bonnie E. Levin, and Gary R. Turner

Financial Exploitation Risk in Older Adulthood: Scope of the Problem

Among older adults, financial loss due to reduced decision-making capacity and increased risk of deception has reached epidemic proportions, constituting an emerging public health crisis. Financial exploitation is now among the most

R. N. Spreng (✉)
Laboratory of Brain and Cognition, Montreal Neurological Institute,
Department of Neurology and Neurosurgery, McGill University, Montreal, QC, Canada

Departments of Psychiatry and Psychology, McGill University, Montreal, QC, Canada

Douglas Mental Health University Institute, Verdun, QC, Canada

McConnell Brain Imaging Centre, McGill University, Montreal, QC, Canada

N. C. Ebner
Department of Psychology, University of Florida, Gainesville, FL, USA

Institute on Aging, Department of Aging & Geriatric Research, University of Florida, Gainesville, FL, USA

Cognitive Aging and Memory Clinical Translational Research Program, University of Florida, Gainesville, FL, USA

Florida Institute for Cybersecurity Research, McKnight Brain Institute, & Pain Research and Intervention Center of Excellence, University of Florida, Gainesville, FL, USA
e-mail: natalie.ebner@ufl.edu

B. E. Levin
Alexandria and Bernard Schoninger Professor of Neurology, University of Miami, Miller School of Medicine, Miami, FL, USA
e-mail: blevin@med.miami.edu

G. R. Turner
Department of Psychology, York University, Toronto, ON, Canada
e-mail: grturner@yorku.ca

R. M. Factora (ed.), *Aging and Money*,
https://doi.org/10.1007/978-3-030-67565-3_5

common forms of elder mistreatment [1–5]. A Senate report released in 2019 found older adults are losing an estimated $2.9 billion annually to financial scams [6]. Other estimates have reached as high as 36 billion [7]. These numbers almost certainly underestimate the actual prevalence of fraud as many older adults are unaware or unwilling to report fraud for fear of appearing cognitively impaired or conforming to negative aging stereotypes [8]. Further, the vast majority of exploitation cases involve family members or close acquaintances and are likely to go unreported or be ignored [1, 9].

These estimates, considered in the context of the rapid expansion of older adults living longer in the United States and other industrialized nations based on projections reported by the Census Bureau, raise concern that financial decision-making deficits in older adulthood will impact an increasingly large segment of the population [5, 10]. Going forward, financial exploitation of older adults is likely to impose increasing societal costs in terms of increasing health care and economic burdens [11]. For older victims of exploitation, experiencing adverse financial events has been associated with greater rates of hospitalization and long-term care admissions, poor physical and mental health, and higher mortality [12, 13]. Older adults acutely feel the effects of financial exploitation, with limited opportunity to recover from loss [14]. Sudden and unexpected financial losses as a result of exploitation may force older adults onto public entitlement systems or relatives to take on unexpected financial burdens. Further, the realization of being a victim of fraud is often accompanied by feelings of self-blame, guilt and embarrassment. These stressors are widely recognized as adversely impacting psychological well-being. However, the specific toll of financial exploitation remains poorly studied and is likely underestimated [15].

At the same time, technological advances are opening up multiple avenues for poor financial decision-making, leading to scams and fraud in our increasingly wired world. In particular, phishing (e.g., via email, text, social media etc.) is a widespread threat and a leading tool for online fraud and subsequent financial exploitation. These attacks are particularly appealing to perpetrators because they are simple, readily available, low-cost to attackers and do not have to occur in mass-scale to be effective. The FBI received 2400 complaints last year with victims' losses from phishing estimated at $325 million [16]. Surprisingly, older adults have largely been neglected in research on cyber-security and online fraud avoidance, even though they may be particularly at risk for such attacks.

Whether in person or online, financial exploitation risk among older adults is emerging as a serious public health concern. These threats will surely increase in the coming decades as the baby boomer generation ages further into older adulthood, taking its place as the wealthiest generation in American history and providing an increasingly lucrative target population for financial fraud. Given the potential scope of the problem, identifying early indicators of financial exploitation risk is critically necessary [17]. In the following sections, we review the cognitive, socio-emotional, and neural determinants of financial exploitation risk that are critically necessary to inform early surveillance efforts. We next present our social cognitive neuroscience model, identifying two pathways to financial exploitation risk in later life. These dual routes to exploitation risk recognize both cognitive and socioemotional factors, as well as the associated neural changes that occur in later life. We close the chapter with a review of financial risk assessment tools, and previewing our work to increase the efficacy of surveillance strategies. Together these efforts are focused toward the ultimate goal of early detection and intervention to reduce the burden of financial exploitation in older adulthood.

Determinants of Financial Risk

Demographic risk factors for financial exploitation include age, lower education, and income levels [18, 19], as well as household size and race [9, 19, 20]. While these demographic factors are important for informing broader policy and public health initiatives, they do not address how to identify a given individual's risk for financial exploitation. Predicting person-specific risk profiles requires a better understanding of individual differences in cognitive and socioemotional capacities, as well as the social and motivational contexts within which financial decisions are made in later life [21, 22]. In a recent review, we proposed a novel model of decision-making in older adulthood incorporating cognitive, socioemotional, and the brain changes associated with the aging process [23]. This model emerged from an earlier survey of the research literature, with particular consideration given to financial decision-making in everyday life, beyond the confines of the laboratory or the clinic. Real-world financial decisions involve weighing concrete choices such as reconciling a weekly budget, managing investment risk profiles, or justifying a big-ticket purchase. Yet we often forget that these decisions are made *in situ,* in complex and shifting social milieu that require navigating emotional reactions and often nuanced social cues. Examples of these *in situ* dynamic social contexts could include the friendly local bank manager who is "recommending" a higher risk (and higher fee) investment portfolio; the insurance telemarketer who calls repeatedly to promote "no medical required" health insurance; or the grandson who continually asks to "borrow" money. Enumerating the scope of financial risks confronting older adults in today's world, from calculating compound interest to calculating complex social agendas and motivations, requires broader consideration of both cognitive and socioemotional capacities. Understanding how these abilities evolve and manifest in the context of age-related alterations in structural and brain function in later life will enable us to define increasingly sensitive risk profiles, improve detection, lessen risk, and ultimately help older adults to avoid fraud and exploitation.

Below we update our review of the recent scientific advances in mapping the cognitive, socioemotional, and neural determinants of altered decision-making in older adults and suggest how these changes may relate to increased financial risk. Yet we urge caution here. It is important not to fall victim to the "aging equals decline" heuristic. The portrayal of older adults as poor decision-makers, vulnerable to exploitation and abuse, continues to propagate through the popular media and in the scientific literature. However, this stereotype has surprisingly mixed empirical support. Older adults often show better or more adaptive decision-making abilities relative to their younger counterparts in many contexts, and these age-related *gains* often manifest in more real-world settings [10]. Over the past decade, the field of decision-science, and more recently, decision-neuroscience [24], has provided a more nuanced picture of the cognitive, affective, social, and neural determinants of decision-making capacity in older adults. Here we take care to highlight both the gains and losses in cognitive and socioemotional functioning that occur throughout older adulthood and how these contribute to differing – but not necessarily declining – financial exploitation risk profiles in later life.

Cognitive changes Cognitive changes in older adulthood have been associated with financial exploitation risk. This has been demonstrated in the context of both age-related cognitive impairments [25, 26] and normative aging [3, 22, 27]. Among the most robust patterns of age-related cognitive decline is a reduction in cognitive control, or "fluid" cognitive abilities. These abilities are necessary to learn novel information, inhibit maladaptive responses, imagine and plan for the future, and to flexibly adapt one's behavior when the decision-making context changes [28, 29]. In the context of financial exploitation risk, age-related declines in cognitive control have been associated with a more risky decision-making style and declines in financial capacity – a critical risk factor for financial fraud and exploitation [18, 30]. Poor cognitive control has been linked to risky decision-making in older adulthood. This risk profile in older adults has been directly associated with greater susceptibility to deceptive advertising, a key tool for fraudsters [31]. Reduced cognitive control capacity has also been associated with poor decision-making, problem-solving, and planning for one's financial future [32, 33]. In addition to these more complex cognitive control abilities, declines in specific cognitive skills necessary for financial transactions have been associated with financial exploitation risk in aging and brain disease [32–34]. Specific cognitive skills that have been investigated in the context of financial management include conceptual, pragmatic, and judgment abilities, ranging from basic (numericity) to more complex skills (financial reasoning and planning). These abilities are necessary to enumerate, allocate, and monitor personal finances in the service of current and future financial goals [34].

However, not all cognitive processes decline with age. Knowledge of oneself and the world, often referred to as "crystallized," conceptual, or semantic knowledge, continues to increase across the adult lifespan, remaining comparatively stable into older age [35]. There is increasing evidence that older adults may be able to draw upon this expanded repertoire of semantic, or fact-based, knowledge to identify potentially fraudulent behavior or avoid exploitative situations [10, 24]. In the context of financial decision-making, Li and colleagues [36] tested this possibility and reported that crystallized cognitive abilities in older adults directly offset losses in fluid abilities, leading to more adaptive financial decisions. Similarly, during a game in which players were required to make financial deals with their fellow game players, older adults rejected more "unfair" offers than their younger counterparts [37]. While younger adults incorporated more empathic responding into their deal-making strategies, older adults tapped into more lived experience (e.g., "money doesn't buy friends") in making their decisions. While the older adults were as empathetic as the young, their reliance on personal experience and prior knowledge to make more "rational" decisions took precedence.

These divergent trajectories of age-related cognitive changes, with fluid cognition decreasing and crystalized knowledge increasing, may also result in a mid-life "sweet-spot" for optimal financial decision-making [38]. While younger adults possess the cognitive control skills necessary to respond flexibly and adaptively to rapidly shifting financial contexts (including the motivations of others), they typically lack the experiential knowledge to identify longer-term patterns and anticipate future consequences. In contrast, older adults have lower fluid cognitive abilities, and reduced financial skills, leaving them vulnerable to exploitation. Yet, they are able to bring more lived experience and prior knowledge to decisions, allowing older adults to more accurately identify and potentially avoid longer-term risk. In the context of these shifting cognitive abilities across the adult lifespan, middle adulthood may provide the optimal balance of executive control and experiential knowledge to maximize financial decisions, in both the near and far terms.

In sum, cognitive changes impact decision-making capacity across the lifespan. These changes have a direct impact on financial competence and magnify exploitation risk for older adults. Fluid cognitive abilities necessary to make complex decisions in uncertain contexts decline. In contrast, greater reservoirs of prior knowledge in later life can be advantageous in contexts where past experience is a reliable predictor of future outcomes. Put simply, the decision-making context matters. Contexts involving speed, pressure, novel information, and shifting contingencies or agendas require high levels of cognitive control and thus leave older adults at greater risk. In contrast, decision contexts that allow for deliberation, and the integration of current facts with prior knowledge, may be particularly advantageous for decision-making in aging.

Socioemotional changes Fraud and financial exploitation, by definition, are transactional, i.e., they involve both victim and perpetrator. Avoiding fraudulent and exploitative or deceptive behaviors depends on the ability to successfully navigate complex, potentially conflict-ridden, social dynamics. In this context, reduced socioemotional capacity would be associated with heightened risk, both for interpersonal exploitation (the grandson who continuously "borrows" money) and for more impersonal, albeit relational, forms of exploitation such as telemarketing fraud [39]. Personal familiarity between victim and perpetrator almost certainly increases the social complexity of potentially exploitative situations. This may be a contributing factor for the overwhelming prevalence of within-family financial abuse [1, 9] and may be further compounded by diminishing social support, loneliness, and a reduced sense of well-being [26, 40, 41].

There is growing evidence that socioemotional factors have different influences on decision-making in older versus younger adults. Older adults show reduced negative emotional arousal to anticipated losses [42]. This absence of negative emotion to anticipated losses suggests that older adults may engage in more risky financial decision-making, and indeed this has been shown to be the case. Older adults make more sub-optimal decisions during risk-seeking (i.e., greater potential for loss), but not during risk-avoidant financial decisions [42]. On a decision-making task designed to mimic real-world shifts in gain and loss contingencies, more than one-third of older adults did not identify altered contingencies and continued to make high-risk decisions [31]. These older participants also failed to show anticipatory emotional arousal during risky choices. This suggests that a significant proportion of older adults may experience a disruption in deception-detection, although the evidence remains somewhat equivocal on this point.

Older adults also demonstrate less reactivity to negative emotional stimuli (see [43] for a review), including explicitly deceptive cues such as lies [44, 45] or breach of financial trust [46]. Reduced arousal to negative emotional cues has been associated with lower activation of a brain region involved in bodily sensation [47]. This may mean that the "gut-feeling" associated with a pending risky decision may be reduced with age [42]. Altered emotional responsiveness to negative stimuli is also consistent with the well-documented "positivity bias" in older adulthood. Older adults show selective attention to, and greater memory for, positively valenced over negatively valenced information (see [48] for a review). In the context of less detailed memories and representations of the future, associated with reduced fluid cognition [49], it has been suggested that older adults may make decisions on the basis of a "bright but blurry" future [50]. Positively skewed, yet less precise, imaginings of the future may heighten the risk of maladaptive long-term decisions.

Age-related emotional changes have direct impacts on decision-making abilities in social contexts, potentially increasing vulnerability to interpersonal exploitation (see [51, 52] for review). For example, older adults assign higher trustworthiness ratings to pictures of unknown faces than do younger adults [47]. They also show reduced flexibility in adjusting financial investment portfolios following a breach of trust by a partner in an investment game. In contrast, younger adults adapted their decision-making style and reduced investments following untrustworthy actions by game partners [46]. Similar age differences in learning the trustworthiness of financial brokers have also been reported [53]. Older adults display positivity biases in other social contexts, including impression formation. For example, they show particular difficulty overcoming positive first impressions such as matching trustworthy faces with untrustworthy behavior [53–56], leaving them vulnerable to potential "wolves in sheep's clothing" [57]. This may pose a particular challenge for older adults encountering the friendly looking, polite con artist who assumes a trustworthy appearance or reputation to mask untrustworthy behavior. It may also present an even greater challenge when assessing the motives of a known other, such as a cherished granddaughter, whose motives for "borrowing" money may change from trustworthy to deceitful over time.

Reduced ability to detect deception in aging has also been demonstrated in the cyber realm, in the context of an ecologically valid field experiment that simulated an e-mail phishing campaign. Older women showed particular vulnerability to a cyber attack [58], and those very old individuals with low cognitive and affective functional profiles were particularly vulnerable [59]. As noted earlier, studies investigating affective influences on decision-making suggest that older adults may adopt a more risky decision-making style in anticipation of a more positively imagined, albeit less detailed, future [50]. These deficits also manifest in the social realm, broadening the specter of vulnerability from maladaptive personal choices to interpersonal exploitation and fraud. Further, age-related changes in socioemotional and cognitive processes likely interact to influence decision-making behavior. These interactions may be positive and beneficial in some contexts. As we described earlier, access to a larger repertoire of prior knowledge has been shown to mitigate impulsive decision-making and reduce temporal discounting during financial decision-making tasks [36]. However, these changes may also compound deficits in more cognitively demanding contexts: older-adult decision-making is particularly impaired on tasks that require rule-learning or shifting contingencies, or involve more abstract or context-dependent reasoning (see [24]), as well as the detection of negatively valenced deceptive cues [44, 46, 58], particularly when cognitive demands are high [60].

Structural and functional brain changes In addition to the cognitive and socioemotional changes outlined above, researchers have examined whether changes in the structure and function of the brain predict financial exploitation risk in normal aging and brain disease. Such changes may provide early biomarkers, signaling increased financial exploitation risk in later life. Early work in this area [61] reported an association between reduced cortical volume in the angular gyrus of the parietal lobe in mild cognitive impairment with performance on a comprehensive measure of financial skills and capacity – the Financial Capacity Instrument (FCI [34]). Performance on the FCI has also been associated with reduced dorsal medial prefrontal cortex volume in early Alzheimer's disease [62]. Together these regions have been implicated in conceptual thinking and the ability to generate a mental image regarding one's future actions [63], two abilities that may be critical for fact-based financial planning, reasoning, and decision-making about monetary allocations.

Appraisal of socially conveyed information in domains relevant to financial exploitation such as deceptive advertising [31, 64], trustworthiness judgments [47, 65], impression formation [56, 66], self other judgments [67], or risky decision-making in novel contexts [68] has been consistently associated with medial prefrontal cortex structure and function. As reviewed briefly above, appraisal of information with high personal significance, or involving social inferences about the actions or intentions of others, is represented more dorsally in medial prefrontal regions, whereas the affective meaning of these contingencies is represented more ventrally [69]. Differences in value expectation have been linked to alterations in an "Affective-Integrative-Motivational" brain circuit, including ventral striatum, anterior insula, medial temporal lobe and prefrontal cortex regions, as well as motor-planning areas [24]. Medial prefrontal cortex is closely connected with limbic structures and ventral striatum, known to mediate affective responses and emotional regulation during decision-making tasks [24]. The integrity of ventral frontal brain regions, and their connections to other brain systems, may be essential for navigating complex social dynamics in situations of high personal relevance, such as potential fraud or exploitation, particularly if the perpetrator is known (see also [52] for a recent extension of the "Affective-Integrative-Motivational" framework to social decision-making in aging).

Dorsal and ventral medial subregions of prefrontal cortex are core nodes in a network of brain regions collectively referred to as the default network [63]. This assembly of functionally connected brain regions is engaged by internally focused thoughts including thinking about one's past, imagining about one's future, or mentalizing about the thoughts or feelings of others [63, 70, 71]. As noted earlier, the majority of financial exploitation incidents are transactional and occur in a social context [1, 9]. Thus age-related brain changes to the default network may predict exploitation risk in older adulthood.

Our work has shown early evidence for this association [72]. We recruited a group of older individuals who had been victims of financial exploitation and a closely matched sample of elderly adults who had been exposed to, but avoided, exploitation. All participants underwent structural and functional brain scans using magnetic resonance imaging (MRI) technology. Older adults who had experienced financial exploitation showed reduced anterior insula volume and increased functional connectivity between this region and the default network (see Fig. 5.1). The anterior insula is a node in the salience network, a collection of brain regions implicated in detecting salient stimuli in the environment [73]. This region has been implicated in generating our "gut-feelings" in potentially deceptive contexts [42, 47] and is also part of the "Affective-Integrative-Motivational" brain circuit associated with decision-making capacity [24]. Increased connectivity between salience and default network brain regions may signal greater reliance on more salient social processing during decision-making in older adulthood. Enhanced salience of social information, combined with altered social processing secondary to default network changes, such as positive impression formation [66], may leave older adults more

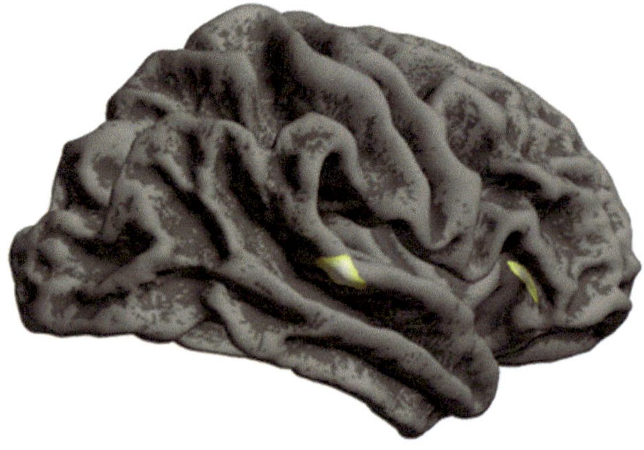

Fig. 5.1 Reduced cortical thickness associated with financial fraud in the anterior insula and superior temporal sulcus/gyrus (right lateral hemisphere)

vulnerable to undue social and affective influences and exploitation. Collectively, these findings suggest that changes in functional connectivity between large-scale brain networks implicated in social decision-making may be an important neural marker of exploitation risk. We explore this idea further in our social cognitive neuroscience model described below (see Fig. 5.2).

In this section, we briefly reviewed the evidence linking age-related changes in cognitive, socioemotional, and neural functions to decision-making ability and financial exploitation risk. Changes in each of these domains, and their interactions, directly influence exploitation risk in older adults. Accurately measuring these changes, and identifying clinically relevant markers of exploitation risk, represents an important next step in early detection and intervention. In the next section, we present our social-cognitive neuroscience model of financial exploitation in older adulthood. This model is intended to provide a framework to guide future research on detection and intervention to reduce the risk of financial exploitation in later life.

Social Cognitive Neuroscience Model of Financial Exploitation

Thus far we have highlighted the cognitive and socioemotional functions that increase vulnerability resulting in poor decision-making ability and ultimately exploitation risk. These include a shift from fluid intellectual abilities to greater reliance on experience and prior knowledge. Other changes include altered socioemotional functioning, including the emergence of a positivity bias, poor sensitivity to future financial loss, reduced deception detection, and poor trustworthiness judgments. Critically, these changes are associated with discrete patterns of functional and structural brain alterations in older adulthood, which in turn may signal context-specific vulnerabilities to financial fraud and exploitation in later life.

We have proposed an integrated social cognitive neuroscience model of financial risk in older adulthood. This model takes into account the complex changes described above as well as their associated neural mechanisms (Fig. 5.2) [23]. We reasoned that addressing the multi-dimensional factors underlying faulty decision-making would yield a more comprehensive framework for developing surveillance and assessment tools. We recognize the myriad determinants driving financial exploitation risk, some of which are fixed such as reading level, socioeconomic status, neighborhood factors, and ethnicity. They also include contextual factors such as financial regulatory regimes, availability of community and social as well as instrumental support, or access to educational and informational resources. However, our model focuses primarily on person-centered factors, such as neuropsychological and functional capacities, as mediated by age-related changes in brain structure and function. Based on the research reviewed above, we identify two behaviorally and neurally distinct pathways to increased financial risk in aging.

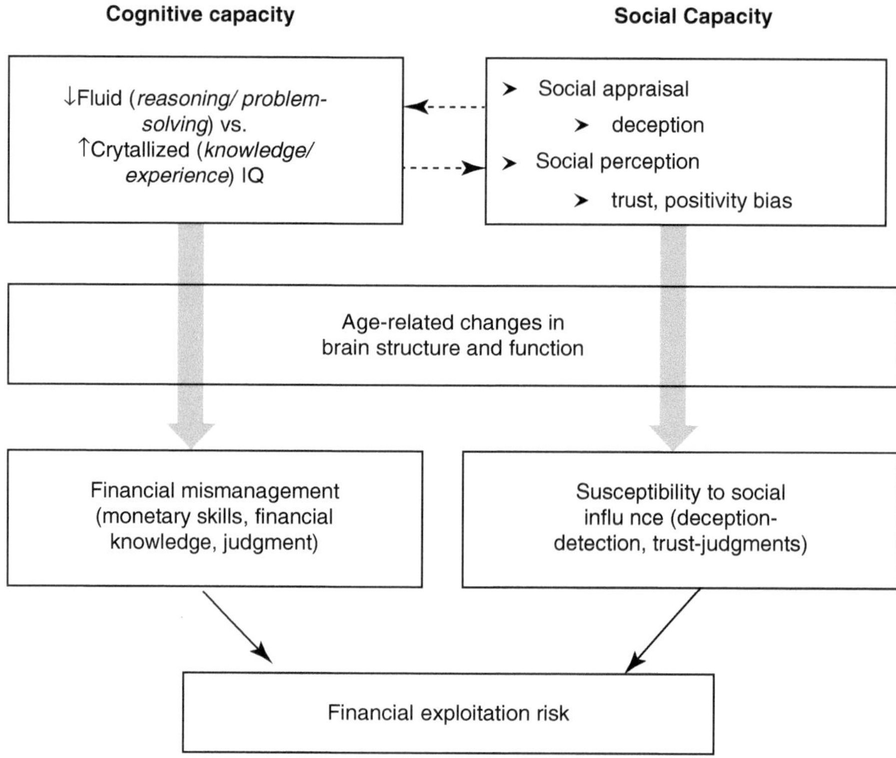

Fig. 5.2 Social cognitive neuroscience model of financial exploitation risk

The first pathway originates from age-related changes in the balance between fluid intelligence abilities (which decline) and crystallized intelligence or prior knowledge (which is preserved). Loss of fluid cognitive abilities may lead to reduced efficiency in maintaining financial goals, inhibiting impulsive behaviors, or flexibly adapting to new contingencies or motivations, whether one's own or those of others. These changes can ultimately result in poor financial decision-making, consistent with past research [18, 41, 74]. The second pathway originates from reduced social capacity (specified in our model as social appraisal and perception) in older adulthood. As reviewed earlier, older adults show reduced ability to appraise and detect potentially deceptive information [31, 46, 58]. They also demonstrate alterations in social perception abilities necessary to make appropriate trustworthiness judgments [55, 56, 64] and display increased attention to more positively valenced information [48]. These changes in socioemotional processing may leave older adults more vulnerable to undue social influences resulting ultimately in increased risk for exploitation at the hands of others, although research directly addressing this relationship remains in its infancy.

Critically, both pathways are associated with dissociable patterns of brain changes in older adults: Functional and structural changes in lateral frontal and parietal brain regions have been implicated in age-related decline in fluid reasoning ability such as working memory, inhibition, and mental flexibility [75], and changes in socioemotional functioning are associated with alterations in the Affective-Integrative-Motivational brain circuit [24], reward circuitry [56], and default network brain regions [61, 64, 66, 72] or their interaction. In developing this social cognitive neuroscience model of exploitation risk in aging, we put forth the idea that recognizing and appreciating these dissociable patterns of behavioral and brain change with age will help in the development of more context-specific indicators of financial exploitation risk in older adulthood (e.g., heightened vulnerability to exploitation in situations of high versus low social complexity).

As depicted in Fig. 5.2, declines in cognitive capacity, associated with changes in lateral prefrontal cortex, would predict increased difficulty with financial management tasks such as problem-solving, planning, or reallocation of resources. In contrast, declines in socioemotional capacities, associated with changes in default network brain regions, or their interactions with limbic regions and subcortical structures involved in affect processing, would lead to increased social vulnerability and exploitation at the hands of others. However, the respective contributions of social and cognitive capacities to social decision-making remain an area of active study [60] and these factors almost certainly interact (represented by the reciprocal arrows in the top row of Fig. 5.2). For example, previous research has shown that declines in working memory are associated with reduced capacity to mentalize about the thoughts or intentions of others [76]. Similarly, working memory for social attributes of others is associated with interactions between default and frontal brain regions [77, 78]. Thus, while there undoubtedly is coupling between social and cognitive capacities at the level of both brain and behavior, the intent of the model is to highlight and emphasize the distinct contributions of cognitive and socioemotional changes to financial risk and how these contribute to context-specific risk profiles for older adults.

Our review thus far has shown that patterns of cognitive and socioemotional functioning, as well as associated brain changes, in later life are well understood. However, adequate surveillance and intervention tools relating to these changes to financial risk profiles do not yet exist. In the next section, we review existing surveillance tools and new directions in assessing financial risk emerging from our own laboratories. These efforts may lead to earlier identification of older adults at risk for financial exploitation, whether through financial mismanagement or undue social influence and coercion.

Financial Risk: Assessment and Surveillance

An array of measures and assessment strategies have been developed to operationalize financial capacity and vulnerability to exploitation in older adults. These include self-report scales such as the Financial Industry Regulatory Authority Risk Meter [79], the Susceptibility to Scams Survey [18], and the Age Associated Financial Vulnerability Survey [40]. Other self-report instruments measure basic skills such as financial literacy, numericity, and planning [80, 81]. More recently, multi-dimensional assessments of financial capacity such as the Lichtenberg Financial Decision Making Rating Scale have been developed [22, 27]. These assess both the contextual (previous history of exploitation and psychological well-being) and intellectual (decision-making capacity) factors that contribute to exploitation risk.

Self-report measures and assessment scales are the most widely available tools for assessing financial exploitation risk. However, comparatively few performance-based measures, necessary for more ecologically valid, in situ assessments, have been developed to measure financial skills and decision-making abilities. Among the most accessible and widely studied of these performance-based measures is the Financial Capacity Instrument (FCI [34]). The FCI was developed as a standardized measure to assess everyday financial skills. It is based on a multi-dimensional construct of financial capacity, encompassing discrete spheres of activity including basic monetary skills, financial conceptual knowledge, cash transactions, checkbook management, bank statement management, and financial judgment. The FCI has been used extensively to quantify declines in financial capacity, as well as providing an early behavioral marker signaling the onset and progression of brain disease [32, 34, 82, 83]. In addition to measuring cognitively dependent financial skills and abilities, our model suggests that performance-based assessments should also incorporate measures of socioemotional functioning. Moreover, these assessments should measure the risk of in-person exploitation as well as risk for the increasingly pervasive incidence of online fraud. Below, we briefly outline our efforts to develop performance-based measures that are able to identify and distinguish cognitive and socioemotional determinants of financial risk, as well as the specific context in which that risk occurs, from personal decision-making to inter-individual exploitation to online fraud.

Structured Assessment of Financial Exploitation Risk (SAFER), developed by Spreng and Turner, is a semi-structured interview based on the Assessment of Capacity for Everyday Decision-making (ACED). The ACED has been used to evaluate decision-making competence in cognitively impaired older adults [84, 85]. We have designed a novel application of the instrument based on our model of financial exploitation risk (Fig. 5.2). This new assessment tool is intended for use in a typically aging population to assess financial decision-making competence, and by extension, exploitation risk. A key feature of the SAFER is the ability to distinguish cognitive and social influences on financial decision-making. During the assessment, older adults are presented with two scenarios, drawn from real cases of financial exploitation. These scenarios were provided and vetted by a local adult protective services office. One scenario involves potential exploitation by an unknown other (credit card telemarketing) and a second involves a known other (theft by a family member). Decision-making competence is assessed along four dimensions: understanding, problem appreciation, reasoning, and decision-making logic. Older adults are asked a series of targeted questions to elucidate their reasoning and rationale for the decisions they make in response to each scenario. Separate scores are computed for decision-making capacity (quality of the response) and content (reliance on social versus non-social information). Early data are consistent with our model. Decision-making competence in these real-world contexts is determined both by the social context and by the cognitive complexity of the decision.

The Assessment of Situational Judgment Task (ASJ), developed by Getz and Levin (under review), examines one's ability to detect scams and infer deception. The ASJ is administered as an online survey and presents scenarios based on FBI cases as well as benign real-life requests for information. Categories of scams include invitations to participate in business opportunities, card skimmers, charity scams, emergency scams, game promotions/sweepstakes, government imposters and deceptive advertisements, identity theft, money transfer/check scams, and online/phishing scams. In addition, subjects are asked to respond to questions pertaining to computer knowledge and scam exposure and experience. This tool was developed for older individuals and includes scams most used against the elderly.

Online fraud susceptibility and cyber security risk assessments Training older adults to avoid online phishing attacks has limited efficacy, as skills are forgotten or poorly applied on the spot. This leaves older adults vulnerable to malicious phishing e-mails, even shortly after training [86]. Based on our field-experimental work that suggested particular vulnerability to e-mail-based phishing among older women [58] and older individuals with low cognitive and affective profiles [59], we identified an urgent need for behavior-based susceptibility profiles to inform intervention and fraud prevention strategies. Toward this goal, we recently developed PEST – the Phishing Email Suspicion Test – an ecologically valid lab-based measure of phishing susceptibility [87]. In PEST, participants rate a series of phishing and non-phishing e-mails regarding their level of suspiciousness. PEST allows quantification of e-mail phishing susceptibility, as participants' overall level of suspicion regarding phishing e-mails and their ability to distinguish phishing from non-phishing e-mails. By comparing suspicion scores for each e-mail to the e-mail's real-world efficacy, we demonstrated the ecological validity of PEST. Phishing e-mails that were more effective in real-world behavior were also more effective at deceiving people in the laboratory. PEST is open-source and can be leveraged in private and corporate contexts to assist in profiling individuals according to their susceptibility risks. Using PEST, we have recently demonstrated reduced ability to discriminate safe from malicious e-mails among cognitively unimpaired older adults [88]. Further, this reduced discrimination ability is more pronounced among older adults at increased genetic risk for cognitive decline secondary to Alzheimer's disease. Using PEST-based individual risk profiling, we are now able to build toward age-tailored/personalized defense solutions. These include decision-supportive monitoring and real-time warnings of potentially deceptive e-mails calibrated to individual risk profiles. Such personalized, automated, real-time cueing offers tremendous potential to assist in the decision-making process and reduce the burden of detecting deception for the individual, with the broader aim to reduce online financial fraud victimization.

Similar initiatives are emerging to provide older adults with information and guidance to reduce victimization in cyberspace. One recent initiative, supported by the Cybercrime Support Network (CSN) in partnership with Google, is ScamSpotter (https://scamspotter.org/). This platform was created to help particularly older adults to avoid getting swindled in the first place by focusing on "three golden rules" (Slow it down, Spot check, and Stop! Don't send) and was designed with seniors in mind to assure user friendliness (e.g., large font size, retro-inspired graphics, and ease of use for mobile devices and social media sharing).

Conclusions and Future Directions

As revealed in this brief review, age-related changes in decision-making capacity can directly influence financial competence and financial exploitation risk in older adulthood. Rapid advances in our understanding of the cognitive, affective, and social determinants of decision-making, and their neural basis, are opening new avenues for identifying person-specific predictors of exploitation risk. However, continued research is urgently needed to narrow the gap between investigations of neural mechanisms underlying decision-making deficits, and assessments of financial competence in the real-world, including cyberspace. The neural mechanisms associated with decision-making, and financial decision-making specifically, in older adulthood are becoming increasingly well defined [24, 89]. This is opening exciting opportunities for the development of more targeted, brain-based decision-making aids. The social cognitive neuroscience framework proposed here (Fig. 5.2) is an important advance in this regard. Our model highlights dual paths to exploitation risk, differentiating cognitive and socioemotional changes and their neural correlates. These two routes to risk may ultimately guide the development of more specific brain and behavioral markers, accounting for the specific contexts, whether in-person or online, in which exploitation is most likely to occur.

Another significant challenge in the field is to bridge the gap between laboratory measures and performance-based, real-world decision-making measures. Efforts are ongoing in this direction, including the development of ecologically valid assessment tools to measure financial competence [34, 84, 85, 90] and online fraud risks [58, 59, 87, 88] in vulnerable older adults. Consistent with our social cognitive neuroscience model, some of these instruments are also being incorporated into a neuroimaging environment to characterize both the brain and behavioral correlates of performance on these tasks [33, 62].

While such advances are essential to mapping the neural and neurocognitive basis of financial exploitation risk, a critical missing link is access to community-dwelling seniors who have been, or continue to be, financially exploited. This is a challenging yet urgently necessary research goal to assess the discriminative validity of measures and markers of exploitation risk. To this end, greater collaboration between the research community and point of care service providers is warranted. Such collaborative efforts are needed to identify older adults who have experienced exploitation for participation in research projects, to vet and validate translational opportunities arising from the research, and ultimately to reinforce this first line-of-defense by providing community and financial services workers with the information and tools necessary to identify and prevent abuse before it occurs.

A White House Council on Aging report urged that much more research be conducted to improve surveillance and early detection of elder abuse [17]. This will require large and diverse samples of older adults who have and have not been victims of exploitation to identify sensitive, specific, and generalizable behavioral and neural biomarkers of exploitation risk that will ultimately be translatable and useful for point of service providers. Large-scale, multi-site, and broadly defined investigations are necessary. As we have shown here, much of this work is well underway. However, efforts need to be rapidly scaled up to match the expanding scope of the problem of financial exploitation risk in our aging population.

References

1. Acierno R, et al. Prevalence and correlates of emotional, physical, sexual, and financial abuse and potential neglect in the United States: the national elder mistreatment study. Am J Public Health. 2010;100(2):292–7.
2. Amstadter AB, et al. Prevalence and correlates of elder mistreatment in South Carolina: the South Carolina elder mistreatment study. J Interpers Violence. 2011;26(15):2947–72.
3. Jackson SL, Hafemeister TL. Risk factors associated with elder abuse: the importance of differentiating by type of elder maltreatment. Violence Vict. 2011;26(6):738–57.
4. FTC. Federal trade commission, consumer sentinal network data book, 2017. Washington, DC; 2018.
5. Burnes D, et al. Prevalence of financial fraud and scams among older adults in the United States: a systematic review and meta-analysis. Am J Public Health. 2017;107(8):E13–21.
6. Aarp. U.S. Senate Aging Committee hearing report on financial fraud. 2019. http://Www.Aarp.Org/Money/Scams-Fraud/Info-2019/Senate-Aging-Committee-Hearing.Html.
7. True-Link. The true link report on elder finanical abuse. San Francisco, USA: True Link Financial; 2015.
8. Pak K, Shadel D. Aarp foundation national fraud victim study. Washington, DC: Aarp; 2011.
9. Peterson JC, et al. Financial exploitation of older adults: a population-based prevalence study. J Gen Intern Med. 2014;29(12):1615–23.
10. Ross M, Grossmann I, Schryer E. Contrary to psychological and popular opinion, there is no compelling evidence that older adults are disproportionately victimized by consumer fraud. Perspect Psychol Sci. 2014;9(4):427–42.
11. Weissberger GH, et al. Physical and mental health correlates of perceived financial exploitation in older adults: preliminary findings from the finance, cognition, and health in elders study (finches). Aging Ment Health. 2020;24(5):740–6.
12. Button M, Lewis C, Tapley J. No victimless crime: the impact of fraud on individual victims and their families. Secur J. 2014;27(1):36–54.
13. Dong X, Simon MA. Elder abuse as a risk factor for hospitalization in older persons. JAMA Intern Med. 2013;173(10):911–7.
14. Nerenberg L. Forgotten victims of elder financial crime and abuse: facing the challenge. J Elder Abuse Negl. 2000;12(2):49–73.
15. Deliema M, Deevey M, Lussardi A, Mitchel OS. Exploring the risks and consequences of elder fraud victimization: evidence from the health and retirement study (December 1, 2017). Michigan Retirement Research Center Research Paper No. 2017-364, Wharton Pension

Research Council Working Paper No. 2018-06. 2017. Available at Ssrn: https://ssrn.com/abstract=3124952 or https://doi.org/10.2139/ssrn.3124952.
16. FBI. Internet crime complaint center, Internet crime report. Federal Bureau of Investigation; 2014.
17. Pillemer K, Connolly M, Breckman R, Spreng N, Lachs MS. Elder mistreatment: priorities for consideration by the white house conference on aging. Gerontologist. 2015;55(2):320–7.
18. James BD, Boyle PA, Bennett DA. Correlates of susceptibility to scams in older adults without dementia. J Elder Abuse Negl. 2014;26(2):107–22.
19. Laumann EO, Leitsch SA, Waite LJ. Elder mistreatment in the United States: prevalence estimates from a nationally representative study. J Gerontol B Psychol Sci Soc Sci. 2008;63(4):S248–54.
20. Beach SR, Schulz R, Castle NG, Rosen J. Financial exploitation and psychological mistreatment among older adults: differences between African Americans and non-African Americans in a population-based survey. Gerontologist. 2010;50(6):744–57.
21. Lichtenberg PA, Ficker LJ, Rahman-Filipiak A. Financial decision-making abilities and financial exploitation in older African Americans: preliminary validity evidence for the Lichtenberg Financial Decision Rating Scale (LFDRS). J Elder Abuse Negl. 2016;28(1):14–33.
22. Lichtenberg PA, et al. Conceptual and empirical approaches to financial decision-making by older adults: results from a financial decision-making rating scale. Clin Gerontol. 2018;41(1):42–65.
23. Spreng RN, Karlawish J, Marson D. Cognitive, social, and neural determinants of diminished decision-making and financial exploitation-risk in aging and brain disease: a review and a new model. J Elder Abuse Negl. 2016;28(4–5):320–44.
24. Samanez-Larkin GR, Knutson B. Decision making in the ageing brain: changes in affective and motivational circuits. Nat Rev Neurosci. 2015;16(5):278–89.
25. Boyle PA, Yu L, Schneider JA, Wilson RS, Bennett DA. Scam awareness related to incident Alzheimer dementia and mild cognitive impairment: a prospective cohort study. Ann Intern Med. 2019;170(10):702–9.
26. Lichtenberg PA. Financial exploitation, financial capacity, and Alzheimer's disease. Am Psychol. 2016;71(4):312–20.
27. Lichtenberg PA, Gross E, Ficker LJ. Quantifying risk of financial incapacity and financial exploitation in community-dwelling older adults: utility of a scoring system for the Lichtenberg Financial Decision-Making Rating Scale. Clin Gerontol. 2020;43(3):266–80.
28. Park DC, Polk TA, Mikels JA, Taylor SF, Marshuetz C. Cerebral aging: integration of brain and behavioral models of cognitive function. Dialogues Clin Neurosci. 2001;3(3):151–65.
29. Schacter DL, et al. The future of memory: remembering, imagining, and the brain. Neuron. 2012;76(4):677–94.
30. Boyle PA, et al. Poor decision making is a consequence of cognitive decline among older persons without Alzheimer's disease or mild cognitive impairment. PLoS One. 2012;7(8):E43647.
31. Denburg NL, et al. The orbitofrontal cortex, real-world decision making, and normal aging. Ann N Y Acad Sci. 2007;1121:480–98.
32. Griffith HR, et al. Impaired financial abilities in mild cognitive impairment: a direct assessment approach. Neurology. 2003;60(3):449–57.
33. Sherod MG, et al. Neurocognitive predictors of financial capacity across the dementia spectrum: normal aging, mild cognitive impairment, and Alzheimer's disease. J Int Neuropsychol Soc. 2009;15(2):258–67.
34. Marson DC, et al. Assessing financial capacity in patients with Alzheimer disease: a conceptual model and prototype instrument. Arch Neurol. 2000;57(6):877–84.
35. Spreng RN, Turner GR. The shifting architecture of cognition and brain function in older adulthood. Perspect Psychol Sci. 2019;14(4):523–42.
36. Li Y, Baldassi M, Johnson EJ, Weber EU. Complementary cognitive capabilities, economic decision making, and aging. Psychol Aging. 2013;28(3):595–613.

37. Beadle JN, et al. Effects of age-related differences in empathy on social economic decision-making. Int Psychogeriatr. 2012;24(5):822–33.
38. Agarwal S, Driscoll JC, Gabaix X, Laibson D. Age of reason: finanical decisions over the life cycle and implications for regulation. In: Brookings papers on economic activity. Washington, DC: Brookings Institute; 2009. p. 51–117.
39. Pinsker DM, Mcfarland K. Exploitation in older adults: personal competence correlates of social vulnerability. Neuropsychol Dev Cogn Section B Aging Neuropsychol Cogn. 2010;17(6):673–708.
40. Lachs MS, Han SD. Age-associated financial vulnerability: an emerging public health issue. Ann Intern Med. 2015;163(11):877–8.
41. Shao J, Zhang Q, Ren Y, Li X, Lin T. Why are older adults victims of fraud? Current knowledge and prospects regarding older Adults' vulnerability to fraud. J Elder Abuse Negl. 2019;31(3):225–43.
42. Samanez-Larkin GR, et al. Anticipation of monetary gain but not loss in healthy older adults. Nat Neurosci. 2007;10(6):787–91.
43. Carstensen LL, et al. Emotional experience improves with age: evidence based on over 10 years of experience sampling. Psychol Aging. 2011;26(1):21–33.
44. Ruffman T, Murray J, Halberstadt J, Vater T. Age-related differences in deception. Psychol Aging. 2012;27(3):543–9.
45. Stanley JT, Blanchard-Fields F. Challenges older adults face in detecting deceit: the role of emotion recognition. Psychol Aging. 2008;23(1):24–32.
46. Frazier I, et al. Age and intranasal oxytocin effects on trust-related decisions: behavioral and brain evidence. Psychol Aging. In press.
47. Castle E, et al. Neural and behavioral bases of age differences in perceptions of trust. Proc Natl Acad Sci U S A. 2012;109(51):20848–52.
48. Charles ST, Carstensen LL. Social and emotional aging. Annu Rev Psychol. 2010;61:383–409.
49. Addis DR, Wong AT, Schacter DL. Remembering the past and imagining the future: common and distinct neural substrates during event construction and elaboration. Neuropsychologia. 2007;45(7):1363–77.
50. Weierich MR, et al. Older and wiser? An affective science perspective on age-related challenges in financial decision making. Soc Cogn Affect Neurosci. 2011;6(2):195–206.
51. Bailey PE, Leon T. A systematic review and meta-analysis of age-related differences in trust. Psychol Aging. 2019;34(5):674–85.
52. Frazier I, Lighthall NR, Horta M, Perez E, Ebner NC. Cisda: changes in integration for social decisions in aging. Wiley Interdiscip Rev Cogn Sci. 2019;10(3):E1490.
53. Rasmussen EC, Gutchess A. Can't read my broker face: learning about trustworthiness with age. J Gerontol B Psychol Sci Soc Sci. 2019;74(1):82–6.
54. Bailey PE, Petridis K, Mclennan SN, Ruffman T, Rendell PG. Age-related preservation of trust following minor transgressions. J Gerontol B Psychol Sci Soc Sci. 2019;74(1):74–81.
55. Suzuki A. Persistent reliance on facial appearance among older adults when judging someone's trustworthiness. J Gerontol B Psychol Sci Soc Sci. 2018;73(4):573–83.
56. Suzuki A, et al. Age-related differences in the activation of the mentalizing- and reward-related brain regions during the learning of others' true trustworthiness. Neurobiol Aging. 2019;73:1–8.
57. Suzuki A, Suga S. Enhanced memory for the wolf in sheep's clothing: facial trustworthiness modulates face-trait associative memory. Cognition. 2010;117(2):224–9.
58. Lin T, et al. Susceptibility to spear-phishing emails: effects of internet user demographics and email content. ACM Trans Comput Hum Interact. 2019;26(5):32.
59. Ebner NC, et al. Uncovering susceptibility risk to online deception in aging. J Gerontol B Psychol Sci Soc Sci. 2020;75(3):522–33.
60. Zebrowitz LA, Boshyan J, Ward N, Gutchess A, Hadjikhani N. The older adult positivity effect in evaluations of trustworthiness: emotion regulation or cognitive capacity? PLoS One. 2017;12(1):E0169823.

61. Griffith HR, et al. Magnetic resonance imaging volume of the angular gyri predicts financial skill deficits in people with amnestic mild cognitive impairment. J Am Geriatr Soc. 2010;58(2):265–74.
62. Stoeckel LE, et al. MRI volume of the medial frontal cortex predicts financial capacity in patients with mild Alzheimer's disease. Brain Imaging Behav. 2013;7(3):282–92.
63. Andrews-Hanna JR, Smallwood J, Spreng RN. The default network and self-generated thought: component processes, dynamic control, and clinical relevance. Ann N Y Acad Sci. 2014;1316(1):29–52.
64. Asp E, et al. A neuropsychological test of belief and doubt: damage to ventromedial prefrontal cortex increases credulity for misleading advertising. Front Neurosci. 2012;6:100.
65. Zebrowitz LA, Ward N, Boshyan J, Gutchess A, Hadjikhani N. Older adults' neural activation in the reward circuit is sensitive to face trustworthiness. Cogn Affect Behav Neurosci. 2018;18(1):21–34.
66. Cassidy BS, Leshikar ED, Shih JY, Aizenman A, Gutchess AH. Valence-based age differences in medial prefrontal activity during impression formation. Soc Neurosci. 2013;8(5):462–73.
67. Ochsner KN, et al. The neural correlates of direct and reflected self-knowledge. Neuroimage. 2005;28(4):797–814.
68. Samanez-Larkin GR, Knutsen B. Reward processing and risky decision making in the aging brain. In: Reyna V, Zayas V, editors. The neuroscience of risky decision making. Washington, DC: American Psychological Association; 2014.
69. Roy M, Shohamy D, Wager TD. Ventromedial prefrontal-subcortical systems and the generation of affective meaning. Trends Cogn Sci. 2012;16(3):147–56.
70. Spreng RN. The fallacy of a "task-negative" network. Front Psychol. 2012;3:145.
71. Spreng RN, Mar RA. I remember you: a role for memory in social cognition and the functional neuroanatomy of their interaction. Brain Res. 2012;1428:43–50.
72. Spreng RN, et al. Financial exploitation is associated with structural and functional brain differences in healthy older adults. J Gerontol A Biol Sci Med Sci. 2017;72(10):1365–8.
73. Uddin LQ. Salience processing and insular cortical function and dysfunction. Nat Rev Neurosci. 2015;16(1):55–61.
74. Han SD, Boyle PA, James BD, Yu L, Bennett DA. Mild cognitive impairment and susceptibility to scams in old age. J Alzheimers Dis. 2015;49(3):845–51.
75. Turner GR, Spreng RN. Executive functions and neurocognitive aging: dissociable patterns of brain activity. Neurobiol Aging. 2012;33(4):826 E821–13.
76. Mckinnon MC, Moscovitch M. Domain-general contributions to social reasoning: theory of mind and deontic reasoning re-explored. Cognition. 2007;102(2):179–218.
77. Meyer ML, Lieberman MD. Social working memory: neurocognitive networks and directions for future research. Front Psychol. 2012;3:571.
78. Meyer ML, Spunt RP, Berkman ET, Taylor SE, Lieberman MD. Evidence for social working memory from a parametric functional MRI study. Proc Natl Acad Sci U S A. 2012;109(6):1883–8.
79. Finra. Financial industry regulatory authority risk meter. Financial Industry Regulatory Authority. 1999, 2020 Online Tool. https://tools.finra.org/risk_meter/.
80. Lusardi A, Mitchell O. Financial literacy and planning: implication for retirement wellbeing. Business Economics; 2007. p. 35–44.
81. Lusardi A, Tufano P. Debt literacy, financial experiences, and overindebtness. National Bureau of Economic Research. NBER Working Paper No. 14808; 2009.
82. Martin R, et al. Declining financial capacity in patients with mild Alzheimer disease: a one-year longitudinal study. Am J Geriatr Psychiatry. 2008;16(3):209–19.
83. Niccolai LM, et al. Neurocognitive predictors of declining financial capacity in persons with mild cognitive impairment. Clin Gerontol. 2017;40(1):14–23.
84. Lai JM, et al. Everyday decision-making ability in older persons with cognitive impairment. Am J Geriatr Psychiatry. 2008;16(8):693–6.

85. Lai JM, Karlawish J. Assessing the capacity to make everyday decisions: a guide for clinicians and an agenda for future research. Am J Geriatr Psychiatry. 2007;15(2):101–11.
86. Caputo DD, Pfleeger SL, Freeman JD, Johnson ME. Going spear phishing: exploring embedded training and awareness. IEEE Secur Priv. 2014;12:28–38.
87. Hakim ZM, et al. Evaluating the cognitive mechanisms of phishing detection with pest, an ecologically valid lab-based measure of phishing susceptibility. In review.
88. Grilli MD, et al. Is this phishing? Older age is associated with greater difficulty discriminating between safe and fraudulent emails. In Review.
89. Samanez-Larkin GR. Financial decision making and the aging brain. APS Obs. 2013;26(5):30–3.
90. Sawrie SM, Marson DC, Boothe AL, Harrell LE. A method for assessing clinically relevant individual cognitive change in older adult populations. J Gerontol B Psychol Sci Soc Sci. 1999;54(2):P116–24.

Chapter 6
Assessing Older Patients' Risk Factors of Being Financially Exploited

Robert E. Roush and Aanand D. Naik

Introduction

Whether physical, psychological, or sexual, or from self-neglect, all forms of elder abuse are especially egregious. Financial abuse and exploitation, is particularly so as the magnitude of losses across the country are staggering, as are the implications to those affected. A study funded by the MetLife Mature Market Institute reported financial losses by exploited seniors a decade ago as almost $3 billion lost annually [1]. Financial losses can result in deleterious effects lasting long after the initial insult to one's dignity and personhood. Other studies suggest that as many as one of five older people is defrauded of money [2, 3] he/she needs to pay for routine living expenses and for out-of-pocket health care costs. Whatever the figure is, it is money no longer working for older Americans, especially in this time of the COVID-19 pandemic of 2020 when businesses and individual portfolios were savaged financially during SARS-CoV-2 outbreaks worldwide. In her April 8, 2020 piece, "Coronavirus Checks: Flattening the Scam Curve," Karen Hobbs of the Federal Trade Commission warns of new ways scammers are pitching fake vaccines and exploiting confusion about the so-called "stimulus checks." Young and older Americans alike may fall for these shameless schemes [4].

Through no fault of their own, some victims of fraud have such health-related conditions as mild cognitive impairment (MCI), dementia, damage to the prefrontal cortex of the brain, and mental health issues. More recent studies have shown low-scam awareness among persons who have yet to exhibit cognitive decline [5] and marked increases in all-cause mortality among those who suffered significant

R. E. Roush (✉)
Baylor College of Medicine, Houston, TX, USA
e-mail: rroush@bcm.edu

A. D. Naik
Professor and Chief, Section of Geriatrics and Palliative Medicine, Department of Medicine, Baylor College of Medicine, Houston, TX, USA

R. M. Factora (ed.), *Aging and Money*,
https://doi.org/10.1007/978-3-030-67565-3_6

monetary losses coined "wealth shock" [6]. Since older people do not have the time to recoup substantial losses, they must often make the difficult choice of foregoing expenses for needed health care. Not receiving those health services or taking their medications and eating properly can hasten a downward spiral, exacerbating often frail conditions that clinicians must then manage. Health care professionals can play a vital role in preventing financial fraud and its consequences by using simple, short, office-based screens to spot the "red flags" in a patient's circumstance that place them at higher risk of financial exploitation.

The genesis of our work on preventing elder financial fraud was an AARP Bulletin article in 2007 based on an interview with the then-US Securities Exchange Commissioner Christopher Cox about his elderly parents having been financially exploited. Both were frail; one had dementia [7]. They were "sold" an unsuitable product resulting in substantial losses that "lined the pockets" of the unscrupulous financial advisor. Mr. Cox decried the fact that the financial losses suffered by his parents hastened their declining health and demise. What emerged from this piece was the thought that, if this could happen to the SEC commissioner's parents, it could happen to any elder. This "sobering" thought led the authors and their colleagues to look into what may be some of the causes of this type of elder abuse.

Since 2009, the "Preventing Elder Investment Fraud and Financial Exploitation" (EIFFE) continuing medical education program has helped train almost 20,000 health care professionals in 32 states, the District of Columbia, and Puerto Rico. The program, funded by the non-profit Investor Protection Trust and Institute, led clinical faculty at Baylor College of Medicine and Harvard University to develop a Clinician's Pocket Guide as the centerpiece of the EIFFE program [8].

Geropsychiatrist Michael Tueth's contributions to preventing elder financial exploitation [9] informs the proposed new arm of the EIFFE program in 2020 that targets the thousands of clinical social workers licensed to provide mental health services to older adults. Acierno et al. (2018) revealed that GAD, depression, and PTSD increase elders' risk of being financially exploited [10]. Furthermore, a 2012 IOM report revealed that 5.6–8 million older Americans – 14–20% of the elderly population – have one or more mental health conditions or problems stemming from substance misuse or abuse [11].

Clinically trained social workers are the nation's largest group of mental health service providers. Social work is considered one of the five core mental health professions by federal law and the National Institutes of Health. With more than 200,000 in the field, there are more clinical social workers than psychologists, psychiatrists, and psychiatric nurses combined. Since the great majority of mental health services in the United States are delivered by clinically trained social workers, it is obvious that these health care professionals be included in the mix of those who treat older adults for the myriad, comorbid, health-related and behavioral conditions they present with [12]. Starting in Texas and with other interested state partners, the next iteration of EIFFE is being planned in conjunction with state chapters of the National Association of Social Workers.

Overview of the Literature

One of the earliest contributors to the body of literature on elder financial abuse was Tueth [9] who wrote about the responsible parties to elder financial fraud, i.e., usually male relative caregivers living with and financially dependent upon the elder in question and who often have mental health and substance abuse issues.

At about the same time, other investigators like Daniel Marson [13, 14] were studying cohorts of persons with dementia and measuring their financial capacity. Marson and his colleagues at the University of Alabama at Birmingham later published results of using their Financial Capacity Instrument to measure cognitive correlates of financial abilities in persons with mild cognitive impairment (MCI). Their findings clearly showed that persons with MCI performed significantly worse than controls, making four times the financial errors than elders without cognitive impairment [15].

Next, University of Iowa neuroscientist Natalie Denburg [16] published her work on persons with and without impaired decision-making. Using the Iowa Gambling Task and neuroimaging, she found that damage to the prefrontal cortex of the brain makes some elders less risk averse, meaning they are more likely to gamble with their money. Denburg suggests that these relatively healthy older adults who make poor decisions are not "demented," but rather they display relatively localized abnormalities in regions of the prefrontal cortex important for exercising good judgment and making complex decisions [17]. Knowing possible causes for damage to this area of the brain – e.g., closed head injuries from auto accidents or falls, repeated blows to the heads of athletes, even severe hypertension – is important to clinicians in advising their patients to take certain precautions.

The first real prevalence numbers for persons with MCI and dementia were published in 2008 by Brenda Plassman at Duke. She found that a full 35% of persons 71 years of age or older had both amnestic and nonamnestic forms of MCI and/or full dementia. At the time of her study, there were over 25 million older adults in that age range, producing almost nine million persons with a major risk factor for financial exploitation [18]. Later MCI prevalence data by Petersen et al. revealed that 40% of persons 75–84 years of age had this early cognitive decline condition [19]. What is so astounding about this epidemiological research is the demographics of an aging population set to almost double by 2030. As the number of older people increases so dramatically, so will those with conditions placing them at risk for financial exploitation [20].

Adding to these prevalence numbers on MCI and dementia is a paper by Bartels and Naslund [21] revealing 5.6 million to 8 million Americans 65 years of age or older with mental health or substance-use disorders. These authors cited an Institute of Medicine estimate that these numbers will increase to 10.1 million to 14.4 million by 2030. They also point to the new Medicare Annual Wellness Visit as a challenge for primary care providers who must screen for depression and cognitive impairment without additional resources and reimbursed time to provide follow-up services. Since depression and other mental health issues can also predispose one to be vulnerable to financial exploitation, the numbers of older adults at risk of losing money they need are even higher than previously thought.

Other estimates of the prevalence of elder financial exploitation range from 5% to 20% [2]. These prevalence rates for financial exploitation are higher than that of systolic heart failure (1–2%), a serious medical condition physicians screen for [22].

The 2011 paper in the *JAMA* by geriatrician Eric Widera et al. on finances in older patients with cognitive impairment made an excellent case of why clinicians should be aware of the issue and screen their patients for vulnerabilities to being financially exploited [23]. Widera and his colleagues in San Francisco rightly pointed out the clinical consequences of a patient's dilemma of having to choose between routine living expenses for shelter, food, utilities, and transportation and unaffordable out-of-pocket costs of needed health care services.

What is so problematic about MCI is individuals can go about living their lives much like they were before: engaged socially, enjoying family, friends, and leisure pursuits; however, those with MCI experience problems with making complex decisions about their financial affairs. Often persons with MCI do not recognize their diminished capacity, nor do spouses or others close to the individual. Until after losses occur; generally, health care providers do not delve into this highly personal area of a patient's life [24].

A major Mayo Clinic longitudinal study tracking the incidence of developing Alzheimer's disease among 1650 normal people of ages 50–70 is being run by Ronald Petersen, MD, PhD. Neuroimaging is being used to determine biomarkers for the spectrum of AD: stage 0 for normal aging and stages 1, 2, and 3 for preclinical, MCI, and dementia, respectively. In addition to neuroimaging and other batteries of tests, Petersen is using Marson's Financial Capacity Instrument to track the continuum of difficulties persons with MCI have in making financial decisions [25].

Petersen and his colleagues at the Mayo Clinic [26] also reported that persons with amnestic MCI have one-year conversion rates to AD from 10% to 15% and that 50% will be diagnosed with dementia within 5 years; thus, it is important to note the date of recorded onset of MCI.

That not everyone who is diagnosed with MCI ever develops full dementia is important to note, especially for the patient and his or her family. And that not everyone who is diagnosed at one point in time with MCI maintains that condition is also important to those with fiduciary responsibilities for the individual. Someone could have MCI from an event such as brain injury, or lack of oxygen during a surgical mishap, or even might have had a previously undiagnosed learning disability that does not worsen with time. Indeed persons with low vitamin B12 levels, thyroid deficiency, or depressive states that have been successfully treated can result in 25% of patients reverting to Petersen's stage zero [27].

What Clinicians Can Do

Widera's strong case for seniors losing enough money to result in adverse health outcomes argues for the dangers of financial fraud being added to an ever-lengthening check list. In PowerPoint slide sets used for the CME programs, an illustration of a prescription pad is shown with check boxes for high blood pressure and blood sugar levels, along with one for vulnerability to financial fraud. When put into the context of health conditions that are routinely assessed in clinical settings, this "prescription for prevention" can be viewed by health care providers and patients alike as something important.

Coupled with the magnitude of the prevalence and the neurobiological basis for seniors' vulnerability to financial exploitation, busy primary care providers and mental health professionals seldom have the time to screen their patients using Marson's gold standard instrument or Denburg's test. Thus, what the authors of this chapter and their colleagues at Baylor College of Medicine in Houston, Texas, have done is to use the science behind the elegant work of others and develop a simple, office-based tool that could reveal "red flags" in a patient's condition that place them at higher risk of being financially defrauded.

Using a structured protocol – the Nominal Group Technique [28] – with focus groups of primary care providers and older persons in Houston, the developers of the EIFFE program sought to devise an unobtrusive method of broaching this hitherto largely unexplored area of patients' lives. Following a series of Round-Robin suggestions, the consensus for an opening interrogatory statement were these two: (1) "In our practice, we find that some people worry about money-related matters. Would you mind if I ask you a few questions?" (2) "I've been reading about elders being financially exploited and thought I'd talk to my mother about her finances, then my own patients, too. May I ask you a question or two about this?" This process of developing an approach to the patient about their finances was not long after the Bernie Madoff scandal made headlines around the world in 2008. Thus, the physician members and elders comprising the focus groups were keenly aware of this issue and interested in our work. Since then, more is known and shared via social media on what seems to be almost daily news about elders being swindled – e.g., the federal Consumer Financial Protection Bureau recently put out an alert that the latest scam was scammers offering to help seniors who lost money to them!

Assessing Patients' Vulnerability to Financial Exploitation

The following information is taken, in part, from a paper submitted by the present authors at the 2012 Annual Meeting of the American Geriatrics Society [29]. In presenting the EIFFE program to the largely clinician audience, geriatrician Aanand Naik made several points relevant to what practitioners can do to screen older patients for their risk of being defrauded. He mainly recommended their use of the Clinician's Pocket Guide. (See at this Web address: http://www.investorprotection.org/downloads/EIFFE_Clinicians_Pocket_Guide_National.pdf.) The guide lists conditions that can be red flags in a patient's history: (a) social isolation, which characterizes many older persons who live alone and whose family members, if they have any, live far away or are inattentive; (b) recent loss of a spouse or adult child and who are continuing to grieve after an extended period of time following that death; (c) dependency upon others for their care and/or providing financial assistance to others; and (d) suffering from substance abuse and/or depression and other mental health issues, as millions of elders do.

If noticeable changes in the patient's cognition, capacity for self-care, fearfulness, appearance, and hygiene are observed, then one can ask such questions as these:

1. Who manages your money day to day? How is that going?
2. Do you run out of money at the end of the month?
3. Do you regret or worry about financial decisions you've recently made?
4. Have you given power of attorney to another person?
5. Do you have a will? Has anyone asked you to change it?

If answers to these questions raise suspicion, you might want to probe deeper by going over the financial checklist in the pocket guide. Ask "Are you having any concerns over the following?" Then read each of the seven items and note how many to which the patient answers "yes."

- I have trouble paying bills because the bills are confusing to me.
- I don't feel confident making big financial decisions alone.
- I don't understand financial decisions that someone else is making for me.
- I give loans or gifts more than I can afford.
- My children or others are pressuring me to give them money or change my will.
- People are calling me or mailing me asking for money, lotteries.
- Someone is accessing my accounts or money seems to be disappearing.

For a global measure of cognitive ability, especially MCI, use the Mini-Cog – a three-item recall and a clock-drawing test as an informational distractor – that can be administered in a primary care provider's office. This three-minute, simple but sensitive test can be downloaded at https://mini-cog.com/ [30]. The full reference for the instrument's developers, Borson et al., is available at https://www.ncbi.nlm.nih.gov/pubmed/11113982, accessed April 27, 2020.

The results of your screen or assessment will likely fall into three categories: (1) normal aging worries about money issues with no particular vulnerability detected; (2) possibly vulnerable enough to warrant referral for further testing or professional assistance with money management; and (3) suspicion that financial exploitation has already occurred requiring mandatory reporting to appropriate authorities.

Referral and Reporting

If a determination is made that a patient may be vulnerable to financial exploitation, then he or she can be referred for such further neuropsych tests as the Financial Capacity Instrument (FCI) described at this link http://knowledge.sagepub.com/view/psychologylaw/n125.xml. Contact information on the developer of the FCI, Daniel C. Marson, PhD, JD, Emeritus Professor at the University of Alabama at Birmingham School of Medicine, Department of Neurology, Division of Neuropsychology, can be obtained at http://www.uab.edu/medicine/neurology/faculty/marson.

If patients consent, they can also be referred to a bonded professional geriatric care manager for assistance who can act as an intermediary with the patient's financial institutions or advisors. Consults with Social Workers and/or calling the United Way 211 hotline (http://www.211.org) may produce local professional care managers or they may also be found by visiting the web site of the Case Management Society of America at http://www.cmsa.org.

If patients need legal advice, they may need the services of an elder law attorney. The local bar association will likely have a list. Others may be obtained from the National Academy of Elder Law Attorneys at http://www.naela.org.

If there's any suspicion that fraud has already occurred, then reporting to Adult Protective Services is required by the laws of most states and grants immunity from civil or criminal liability for professionals who report suspected cases of abuse. To find your state's APS contact to make confidential reports, use this link: https://www.napsa-now.org/get-help/help-in-your-area/.

If the nature of the financial exploitation involves a stock broker or financial advisor, then the securities regulators in one's state should be contacted, as they will investigate to see if an unsuitable financial product has been sold to the elder in question. Suitability takes into account one's capacity to understand the product and its risk, the individual's age, and the size of the person's financial portfolio. Reputable brokers will know these characteristics of a client. To locate the Securities Office Regulators in your state, visit the North American Securities Administrators Association at http://www.nasaa.org. No health care professional will violate patient privacy as protected by HIPAA if the reporting physician only gives the patient's name and contact information. The attorneys in the state securities offices will treat the reported information confidentially.

Other types of financial fraud are often perpetrated, e.g., unsuitable annuity contracts sold by insurance agents and unscrupulous real estate agents who undervalue an elder's property and then use undue influence to buy it and flip it for a profit. This type of fraud can also be reported to state agencies overseeing the licensing and practices of insurance and real estate agents and brokers. And any theft by fraud can and should be reported to the local district attorney's office.

Following are the final points on managing the older patients who present in your office or clinic:

1. Be particularly observant of who accompanies the elder to the medical office. If that person seems overly protective and dominant, utters demeaning remarks about the patient, is anxious to leave, and/or threatens to take the patient to another physician or clinic, then the possibility of elder abuse should be suspected and acted upon.
2. In exercising your duty, perhaps conclude the discussion with your patients of who is managing their money and how that is going with these admonitions: Be aware of your vulnerability. Be aware of who wants your money. Be aware of how you can protect yourself. Be aware of who can help you.
3. Given the demographic and epidemiological data on aging persons, consider the value of making earlier than usual screening for cognitive impairments that may lead to actionable diagnoses. Support for this are data on how early-stage AD adversely affects household financial outcomes. Gresenz et al. point to their findings being consequential because financial vulnerability during the disease's early stage could greatly impact the ability of afflicted individuals and their families to pay for care in the later stage [31].

And, in an interesting play on words, "whealthcare" will be achieved when financial services and health care professionals accept their collective responsibility to support their client-patients' wealth and health [5]. Given all we know about the relationship of socio-economic status and access to health care, it would seem incumbent on all those who have a fiduciary responsibility for an elder, especially one with MCI or other neurodegenerative conditions, to collaborate in the protection of those they serve.

Finally, tell your patients that you are concerned about financial exploitation and to be careful in whom they place their trust. And, as there's no such thing as a "free lunch or dinner," when asked to attend one of these functions or when receiving a call from someone you don't know, politely hang up!"

EIFFE and Investor Education Resources

One can obtain all the educational materials produced by the EIFFE Prevention Program including the Clinician's Pocket Guide, a Patient Education Brochure, and short video clips that depict the plight of older persons victimized by financial fraud by going to the Investor Protection Trust web site http://www.investorprotection.org/ipt-activities/?fa=eiffe-pp. Also, at this site, a free, one-hour CME program for Category I Credit in Medical Ethics is being developed. For more general investor education resources, peruse the remainder of the IPT site.

Authors' Notes and Acknowledgments The present authors (Roush and Naik) gratefully acknowledge their colleagues and funders of the EIFFE program. Without their contributions and support, the program would not have been possible.

Jennifer A. Moye, PhD, is a geropsychologist at the VA Boston Healthcare System and Professor, Department of Psychiatry, Harvard Medical School. Whitney L. Mills, PhD, is a Health Services Research Postdoctoral Fellow with the Houston Health Services Research & Development Center of Excellence at the Michael E. DeBakey VA Medical Center in Houston, TX. Mark E. Kunik, MD, Professor of Psychiatry, is also at the Michael E. DeBakey VA Medical Center. Nancy L. Wilson, LMSW, is a Faculty Associate at Baylor's Huffington Center on Aging. George E. Taffet, MD, is former Chief of the Section of Geriatrics, Department of Medicine (the position now held by his successor, Aanand D. Naik, MD), Baylor College of Medicine. Justin P. Wheeler, B.S., was Assistant Project Director, Huffington Center on Aging and Texas Consortium Geriatrics Education Center.

This work was supported by grants from the Investor Protection Trust (the 2009–2010 Texas project) and the Investor Protection Institute for the subsequent coalition of 32 states and jurisdictions for the 2011–2020 project. Both projects benefitted from funding to Baylor's Texas Consortium Geriatric Education Center provided by the federal Health Resources and Services Administration. The former TCGEC was headed by Dr. Roush from 1985 to 2016. The present HRSA-funded project that remains focused on elder abuse is the Southeast Texas GWEP (Geriatrics Workforce Enhancement Program) headed by Dr. Naik and Angela Catic, MD, M.Ed., who directs the Baylor Geriatrics Fellowship Program.

Grateful appreciation is extended to Mr. Don Blandin, former President and CEO of the Investor Protection Trust and the Investor Protection Institute, and to Ms. Cheri Meyer, Senior Vice President, plus all the investor educator professionals in the various state securities offices who, along with the clinical presenters at the many CME events, made this project possible.

References

1. MetLife Foundation. The MetLife study of elder financial abuse: crimes of occasion, desperation, and predation against America's elders. New York: Metropolitan Life Insurance Company; 2011.
2. Acierno R, et al. Prevalence and correlates of emotional, physical, sexual, and financial abuse and potential neglect in the United States: The National Elder Mistreatment Study. Am J Pub Health. 2010;100(2):292–7.
3. Infogroup/ORC. Elder investment fraud and financial exploitation: a survey conducted for Investor Protection Trust. 2010 http://www.investorprotection.org/downloads/pdf/learn/research/EIFFE_Press_Release.pdf. Cited March 20, 2012.
4. Hobbs K. (April 8, 2020) Coronavirus Checks: Flattening the Scam Curve. Retrieved April 23, 2020 from https://www.consumer.ftc.gov/blog/2020/04/coronavirus-checks-flattening-scam-curve.
5. Karlawish J. Social cognition and the aging brain. Ann Intern Med. 2019:1–2. https://doi.org/10.7326/M19-0907.
6. Garber AM. From misfortune to mortality, sudden loss of wealth and increased risk of death. J Am Med Assoc. 2018;319(13):1327–8. https://doi.org/10.1001/jama.2018.3418.
7. Magnusson P. New head of the SEC: swindlers besieged Christopher Cox's parents. Now, as SEC chairman, he's fighting back. AARP Bulletin. 2006;47(2):31–4.
8. Roush RE, Moye JA, Mills WL, Kunik ME, Wilson NL, Taffet GE, Naik AD. Why clinicians need to know about the elder investment fraud and financial exploitation program. Generations. 2012;36(2):94–7.
9. Tueth MJ. Exposing financial exploitation of impaired elderly persons. Am J Geriatr Psychiatry. 2000;8:2.
10. Acierno R, Watkins J, Hernandez-Tejada M, Muzzy W, Frook G, Steedley M, Anetzberger G. Mental health correlates of financial mistreatment in the National Elder Mistreatment Study

Wave II. J Aging Health. 2019;31(7):1196–211. https://doi.org/10.1177/0898264318767037, Epub 2018 Apr 17

11. Institute of Medicine. The mental health and substance use workforce for older adults: in whose hands?. Washington, D.C.: The National Academies Press; 2012. Retrieved April 28, 2020 from https://doi.org/10.17226/13400.
12. GoodTherapy. (December 14, 2015). The Important Role Social Workers Play in Mental Health. Retrieved April 28, 2020 from https://www.goodtherapy.org/blog/the-important-role-social-workers-play-in-mental-health-1214157.
13. Marson D. Loss of financial capacity in dementia: conceptual and empirical approaches. Aging Neuropsychol Cogn. 2001;8:164–81.
14. Marson DC, et al. Clinical interview assessment of financial capacity in older adults with mild cognitive impairment and dementia. J Am Geriatr Soc. 2009;57:806–14.
15. Okonkwo OC, Wadley VG, Griffith HR, Ball K, Marson DC. Cognitive correlates of financial abilities in mild cognitive impairment. J Am Geriatr Soc. 2006;54(11):1745–50.
16. Denburg NL, et al. The orbitofrontal cortex, real-world decision-making, and normal aging. Ann NY Acad Sci. 2007;1121:480–98.
17. Denburg NL, Harshman L. Why so many seniors get swindled: brain anomalies and poor decision-making in older adults. 2009. http://www.dana.org/news/cerebrum/detail.aspx?id=23106. Retrieved March 20, 2012.
18. Plassman BL, Langa KM, Fisher GG, Heeringa SG, Weir DR, Ofstedal MB, et al. Prevalence of cognitive impairment without dementia in the United States. Ann Intern Med. 2008;148(6):427–34.
19. Petersen RC, Lopez O, Armstrong MJ, et al. Practice guideline update summary: mild cognitive impairment: report of the guideline development, dissemination, and implementation Subcommittee of the American Academy of Neurology. Neurology. 2018;90(3):126–35. https://doi.org/10.1212/WNL.0000000000004826. Epub 2017 Dec 27
20. Karp N, Wilson R. Protecting older investors: the challenge of diminished capacity. Washington, D.C.: AARP Public Policy Institute; 2011.
21. Bartels SJ, Naslund JA. The underside of the silver tsunami – older adults and mental health care. N Engl J Med. 2013;368:493–6.
22. American Heart Association. Heart disease and stroke statistics. Dallas (TX): American Heart Association. 2009:20. Available from: http://www.nanocorthx.com/Articles/HeartDiseaseStrokeStatistics.pdf.
23. Widera E, Steenpass V, Marson DC, Sudore R. Finances in the older patient with cognitive impairment: He didn't want me to take over. J Am Med Assoc. 2011;305(7):698–706.
24. Moye J, Marson DC. Assessment of decision-making capacity in older adults: an emerging area of practice and research. J Geron Psych Sci. 2007;62:P3–P11.
25. Petersen RC. Neuroimaging and biomarkers: How early can we diagnose Alzheimer's disease? Robert Butler, MD, Memorial Lecture, National Institutes of Health 2013 May 8; Bethesda MD.
26. Petersen RC, Smith GE, Waring SC, Ivnik RJ, Tangalos EG, Kokmen E. Mild cognitive impairment: clinical characterization and outcome. Arch Neurol. 1999;56(3):303–8.
27. Anderson ND, Troyer AK, Murphy KJ. Mild cognitive impairment: the border zone between cognition and dementia. Aging Today. 2012 Nov-Dec:4.
28. Delbecq AL, VandeVen AH. A group process model for problem identification and program planning. J Appl Behav Sci. 1971;7:466–91.
29. Factora R, Naik AD, Roush RE, Ulrey P. Truth and consequences: Mickey Rooney, geriatric assessment, and risk for financial exploitation. Annual Meeting of the American Geriatrics Society; 2012 May 3; Seattle, WA.
30. Borson S. The mini-cog: a cognitive "vital signs" measure for dementia screening in multilingual elderly. Int J Geriatr Psychiatry. 2000;15(11):1021.
31. Gresenz CA, Mitchell JM, Marrone J, Federoff HJ. Effect of early-stage Alzheimer's disease on household financial outcomes. Health Econ. 2019;29(1):1–12. Accessed May 30, 2020 from https://onlinelibrary.wiley.com/toc/10991050/2020/29/1.

Chapter 7
Clinical Assessment of Financial Decision-Making Capacity

Ronan M. Factora

An 84-year-old man arrives in the clinic with his daughter. She is concerned that her father has been becoming more forgetful and often finds she has to repeat herself multiple times. Recently, he gets ready for social events, such as dinner, early in the morning, and usually after being told that they were going to go out in the evening. His bank account seems to be suffering as well, and she has been finding a number of bills and documents in his mail from companies she knows he didn't have business relationships with before.

Introduction

As older persons make up a larger proportion of the world population, they present an increasing percentage of the wealth pool. Between 2010 and 2050, the US population over the age of 65 is expected to more than double, from 40 million to 88 million [1]. Medical professionals represent one group that has almost ubiquitous exposure to the aging population. With increasing chronic disease burdens, most persons over the age of 65 will be exposed to doctors. Over 92% of patients with Medicare coverage will have seen a physician in the last year [2]. Therefore, it could be considered that one of the best opportunities for detection of financial exploitation lies within the healthcare system. Efforts to increase awareness of elder mistreatment and financial exploitation among physician providers have been of paramount concern to a number of nongovernmental organizations. Efforts currently focus on educating physicians in the assessment of financial decision-making capacity (FDMC).

R. M. Factora (✉)
Cleveland Clinic Lerner College of Medicine at Case Western Reserve University, Cleveland Clinic, Cleveland, OH, USA
e-mail: factorr@ccf.org

R. M. Factora (ed.), *Aging and Money*,
https://doi.org/10.1007/978-3-030-67565-3_7

When discussing the issue of decision-making capacity, this typically refers to the individual's ability to do the following: understand their current situation (social, financial, medical), be able to understand why the choice needs to be made (consequence), the types of choices that can be made, and the ability to definitively make a choice [3]. From a financial perspective, this means understanding why the decision needs to be made and what the impact of that transaction will have on their financial situation. For purposes of clarity, the term "competence" will be avoided. In some jurisdictions "competence" is a legal term connoting that a person's decision-making capacity has been ruled on by a court. Though the terms "competence" and "capacity" are often connected, and in some areas are used interchangeably, often a court will ask for a medical professional's opinion as to the decision-making capacity of a person before ruling on their competence. Additionally, impaired decision-making capacity in one area should not lead to the conclusion that that same individual lacks the capacity to make decisions in other areas. As there are many areas where decision-making capacity can be determined (financial, medical, testamentary, etc.), the discussion in this chapter will focus specifically on financial decision-making capacity.

The Clinician's Dilemma

Medical professionals experience great difficulty in ascertaining the financial decision-making capacity (FDMC) of older persons. Overall, these attitudes seem to stem from personal discomfort in asking patients about financial matters based on a fear that such questions violate physician-patient trust. To counter such attitudes, it may be useful to remind providers that such discussions are similar to discussions of end-of-life issues and advance directives – uncomfortable but necessary. Additionally, since FDMC is closely related to cognitive impairment [4], avoiding the topic of a person's ability or inability to independently manage their financial affairs (as part of the evaluation of functional status of older persons) may prevent further identification of functional impairments (which could uncover a diagnosis of dementia). One small study has put the rate of failure to diagnose dementia as high as 65% [5].

Screening for FDMC

Impaired FDMC may be due to a number of both cognitive and affective disorders; these disorders may include dementias, late effects of cerebrovascular disease (stroke), and depression. Though a discussion about evaluation of cognitive impairment is beyond the scope of this chapter, screening for impairment in FDMC can start with the simple question of "Who manages your finances for you?" An answer that is in disagreement with what is reported by the caregiver or other close friend or family member (who can provide collateral information about that individual's functional status or report observed problems with that person's ability to manage their finances) may be a good sign that a problem with FDMC may be present. Responses indicating that an individual is managing their own finances can be followed up by questions of what bills are being paid regularly and are there any problems with balancing the checkbook – questions that are meant to convince the interviewer that this person is likely managing their affairs independently and appropriately. If the individual identifies another person as the responsible party for managing their finances, it is worthwhile to ask the reason why another person is managing their finances. This line of questioning helps reveal if the person being interviewed has recognized that they were in fact having difficulty managing their financial affairs and has proactively sought out assistance to ensure that their financial affairs are in order. These questions may also reveal who is currently managing the finances, if the person being interviewed trusts them, what time frame this person was assigned this responsibility, and if there are any concerns from the person being interviewed about how this surrogate decision-maker is executing their responsibilities.

Another commonly used question that may identify an issue is "Have you noticed any unusual transactions in your bank account?" This question focuses on the possibility of financial exploitation in the patient suffering from impaired FDMC. A lack of awareness of where monies are directed or lack of ability to explain why certain financial decisions are made (unexplained high costs of services, multiple payments of the same bill, opening of new accounts/loans/credit cards, etc.) may be a sign that this individual is at risk for exploitation or is already frankly being exploited. Sometimes concerns about difficulty managing finances or concerns about the types of transactions being conducted may come from those who know the person being interviewed. In fact, observations from family, friends, and other members of the community are often the first sign that problems are present.

Red Flags

Often, the chief complaint at an office visit may give hints to a possibility of FDMC impairment. These "red flags" also may indicate that a primary disease condition, such as a dementia, may be the cause of impairment. FDMC can be assessed by both observable and subjective features. Paying attention to a person's state of dress, ability to pay clinic bills, or evidence of new neurologic deficits are helpful in determining if there has been a functional change. Subjective features are often volunteered by caregivers or relatives, who will often notice unusual behaviors that could indicate cognitive decline. While not as common, patients themselves may offer their own concerns of being financially exploited. Some typical behavioral changes that can also be associated with impaired FDMC include [3]:

1. Decline in personal hygiene
2. Paranoid (accusatory) behavior about "theft" of money or possessions
3. Erratic or unusual financial transactions

4. Increased "gifting" of personal possessions
5. Obsession with misinterpreted financial statements

The challenge to the clinician may be in determining whether accusations of theft or an unusual pattern of transactions may have a basis in purposeful fact. In such situations, excluding the possibility that this person *is* the victim of theft should be pursued before proceeding with the conclusion that this individual is experiencing a paranoid delusion. A simple way to clarify this is to ask the individual details about the event, including how much money (or what items) have been stolen – the details that are offered may provide some insight that the individual may have been experiencing a delusion. In dementia, the amounts usually are not able to be recalled ("lots" instead of an actual figure). In psychotic disorders, the amount of money stolen may be incredibly high ("millions") and items stolen likewise incongruous with reality. Some examples include accusations that others have stolen the fillings of their teeth, the insulation from their home, and vital organs. It is always a good idea to follow up *any* screening question or red flag with a request for specifics.

Collateral information from family, friends, and caregivers may also help substantiate or counter the offered claims. Differences in the explanations provided by the family/friends/caregivers and the patient have to be explored, often with the content of each person's details and the results of cognitive testing leading to favoring one version over another. If there is uncertainty about whether or not statements regarding exploitation or theft are correct, involvement of community agencies such as Adult Protective Services can lead to investigation of such claims.

Dementia and FDMC

Dementia is (at its core) a loss of cognitive function that is severe enough to interfere with a person's functional status. In some circumstances, executive function may be affected. The consequence may be impairment in an individual's ability to create, understand, and execute plans to handle financial tasks, making financial abilities such as balancing a checkbook, paying bills, managing investments, or negotiating terms for loans or other complex financial transactions very difficult. Though attempts may be made by the individual to perform these tasks independently, evidence of difficulty may be seen in frequent omissions or duplication of transactions. A commonly encountered scenario in the clinic might involve a family member voicing concern that their loved one fails to pay bills, or writes a check twice for the same bill, leading to utilities being cut off, vehicles being repossessed, or even having a residence foreclosed.

In dementia, impairment in function (including the ability to manage finances) may already be evident. Prior to this point, there is a spectrum of cognitive decline and impairment that may be associated with an increase in the risk for making poor financial decisions. Increasing cognitive impairment is associated with a greater risk of financial exploitation. This period of increased risk precluding clinical dementia may for last years. Persons in this situation may experience a reduced ability to assess risk and recognize "untrustworthy" persons. One study identified the unusual "advantage" the untrustworthy person has; older persons with cognitive changes are more likely to remember an untrustworthy face rather than a trustworthy one and are more likely to judge an untrustworthy face as one that is more trustworthy [6] – hence, these individuals may remember the face of the untrustworthy individual (rather than the trusted individual) but may not recognize them as untrustworthy. Older persons without cognitive impairment are usually not affected in such a way and have relatively equal risk taking performance when compared to younger persons [7]. Chapter 5 by Dr. Spreng and his colleagues reviews this topic in detail and discusses the complexities underlying decision-making capacity (specifically focusing on vulnerability of older persons to this risk) and also briefly reviews tools that could be useful in assessing financial risk.

There is a predictable decline in financial decision-making capacity as dementia advances. During these periods, there is a transition from dysfunction of planning and organization to frank loss of the ability to calculate sums and perform basic mathematical calculations essential in managing finances. The result is an inability to subtract a sum of money from a larger balance and often an inability to do simpler transactions such as making change. This is partly caused by the inability to remember the "steps" involved in making change – total balance minus spent amount equals remaining balance. The ability to execute complex sum calculations can be lost in the mild stage, but in the moderate stage, the ability to calculate simpler sums of 1–2 digit sizes is affected.

An additional impacted area is the loss of abstract thinking. As the value of money is an abstract concept to most individuals at this stage of dementia, this impairment results in the inability to correlate an amount being spent with the value of a product purchased. For example, if asked "what kind of item costs $10,000?", a person at this stage is unlikely to come up with an appropriate answer or may confabulate one. An example of one common vague answer may be "a lot of things. Following this question up with the reverse, such as "how much does a loaf of bread cost," may result in a similar response (answers are usually a multiple of an even number). This loss of correlation with "value" and "cost" may impair an individual's ability to recognize the true costs of items purchased or services being offered. Scams of at-risk individuals arise from this impairment, with victims falling prey to excessive charges for services for simple home repairs or requests to pay exorbitantly high prices for basic items.

When a person suffering from dementia has a caregiver, many of these deficits are often concealed or compensated for by the financial assistance provided by the caregiver. Often there is an unmasking of financial incapacity when that caregiver (often a spouse) dies or suffers significant impairment. Direct questions regarding the patient's capacity may have been dismissed by the former caregiver, but when a new one takes over (such as a child), new light is often shed on the degree of impairment.

Risk Assessment of Financial Decision-Making Capacity

Identifying FDMC is often dependent on diagnosing and correctly staging dementia. Many tools exist to help achieve this goal, but time constraints may limit a physician's ability to utilize them in practice. The Mini-Cog is a quick tool that can often help identify patients that may require more in-depth testing. The test consists of two queries: (1) the patient is given three words, asked to repeat them to make sure they are understood, and then is asked to recall them a brief time afterwards, and (2) in between the parts of the recall, the patient is asked to draw a clock (placing all 12 numbers in the circle and then placing the hands at a the time of ten past eleven). Scores are based on performance of the two queries. Cognitive impairment is diagnosed if the patient cannot recall any of the three words or if they can recall less than three but have an abnormal clock drawing test. This test usually takes 3 minutes to perform [8].

Another test that helps focus on FDMC is found in the Saint Louis University Mental Status Exam (SLUMS). Question 7 on the test is a simple change calculation problem:

You have $100 and you go to the store and buy a dozen apples for $3 and a tricycle for $20.

1. *How much did you spend? (1 pt.)*
2. *How much do you have left? (2 pts.)*

A score of 3 on this section suggests that the simple task of calculating cost and making change is intact – essential functions for simple financial transactions. A score of 1 or 0 suggests impairment of the ability to perform those transactions and may indicate the presence of greater impairment in FDMC. Completion of the entirety of the SLUMS may help reveal the extent and severity of cognitive impairment and is worthwhile when confronted with a complaint of memory loss or suspicion of dementia. This quantitative measure could provide useful information if determination of competence by the court is pursued [9, 10].

The third test is "serial 7s" – an exercise where the patient is asked to count backward from 100 in intervals of "7" (93, 86, etc.) for five intervals. Difficulty executing this task may demonstrate not only problems with mathematical function but also in memory and concentration. This task was popularized by the Folstein "Mini Mental Status Exam" [11] and incorporated also in the Montreal Cognitive Assessment (MoCA); however it is more difficult than the change questions in the SLUMS. Regardless of which test that is chosen, preference would lean toward those involving calculation and planning, as these are two core requirements for FDMC. Impairment in these domains would support suspicion of impaired FDMC.

For the court to determine financial competency, the above testing and a clinician's statement discussing the results are often sufficient; however, further testing (such as a longer neuropsychiatric battery, including measures of executive function, problem-solving, and memory, or the use of validated tests for financial decision-making capacity) is advised to more accurately assess the extent and severity of the cognitive impairment. Regardless of the test results, it is necessary to correlate findings of impairment with real-world documentation of that person's inability to manage finances (such as late bill payments, overdrafts, inability to manage balances, documentation of victimization to fraud/exploitation). The combination of (1) impaired cognitive function (through the testing suggested above) and/or identification of impairment financial decision-making capacity utilizing validated tools with (2) documented inability of that individual to appropriately manage their financial affairs should support a finding that this individual truly lacks the ability to make independent financial decisions and consequently should be assigned an alternative means of ensuring that their financial affairs are managed appropriately and in a manner directed at that person's best interests.

Mitigation of Risk

After determining if there is cognitive impairment and/or impaired FDMC, stabilization of that individual's financial status should be the goal. In some circumstances, assignment of durable power of attorney (DPOA) for finances may be enough to protect the individual's financial interests, with that designated person given the authority to carry out financial transactions for this individual in question. Arranging a DPOA is one important step in making sure that trusted individuals are granted access and authority to help manage financial affairs. Such decisions and drafting of documents ideally should take place before any significant cognitive impairment develops (see Chap. 14). While drafting of a DPOA may be acceptable in mild cognitive impairment and early dementia, its legal status can be challenged if the document is drafted when that individual has more advanced cognitive impairment or dementia (particularly if there is any suggestion that the patient had impairment in his/her ability to understand the consequence of completing the DPOA). In essence, once the patient loses the capacity to identify a surrogate decision-maker for finances, it may be too late to have them sign a DPOA document.

If DPOA is not possible to be arranged due to impaired cognitive function, then applying for conservatorship of finances could be an alternative intervention. A petitioner, usually a family member, could submit an application to the appropriate legal authority (in most US jurisdictions, this is handled by the probate court). This is often an uncontested process; however if financial exploitation is occurring within the family, the offending party will often attempt to block an assignment of this authority.

Assignment of guardianship is the ultimate legal remedy to impaired decision-making capacity. The guardian is given the authority and responsibility by the court to ensure that financial decisions are made in the best interests of the person deemed "incompetent" and is typically granted access to all of that individual's financial accounts and assets in order to achieve this goal. Less restrictive solutions should be considered first prior to pursuing this solution (as detailed above), but many times, assignment of a guardian under law is necessary to ensure that financial decisions are made appropriately, particularly if the individual involved continues to make poor financial decisions for themselves despite the presence of DPOA or conservator.

In any circumstances where a surrogate decision-maker is activated to make decisions for the person in question, it should also be determined that this surrogate is also capable of executing the responsibilities associated with the authority granted. The following examples highlight some of the dilemmas that may be faced in situations where surrogate decision-makers are involved.

Example 1

A 74-year-old woman with a history of atrial fibrillation presents with her husband, who is concerned that his wife is having trouble with handling finances. She suffered a stroke 3 months ago, and while she does not seem to have any motor deficits, she has developed unusual speech habits. Her husband states she often stops mid-sentence, trying to remember words, and will get frustrated – even angry – if she cannot recall them. She also sometimes confuses the names of items, such as calling a chair a "stove." While previously able to manage the household finances, her husband has had to assume control, even hiring a financial advisor to help organize their retirement and investment accounts.

Discussion

Cognitive impairment can also occur in conditions other than neurodegenerative disorders such as Alzheimer's disease. In practice, patients who have suffered cerebral infarcts in the territory of the middle cerebral artery (such as from cardiac thromboemboli in atrial fibrillation) will often develop aphasia/expressive language impairment. In this case, while the infarct spared motor functions, it affected linguistic areas. While expressive aphasia (such as this patient's) often do not indicate impaired FDMC, its presence may also be associated with increased likelihood that other infarcts may have occurred, impairing other areas of cognition and function. In this case, it is the *husband's FDMC* that should be assessed since he is now assuming care of the finances due to his wife's stroke. Since he is also using a financial advisor, his risk of being financially exploited now increases. Validity of any DPOA is dependent on the DPOA's decision-making capacity.

Example 2

A 67-year-old man who lives alone has recently been diagnosed with medication-refractory depression and is now undergoing electroconvulsive therapy (ECT). After several treatments, it becomes clear that he is developing significant post-procedure amnesia, and while the depression is apparently improving, his ability to care for himself has now come into question. This week, the clinic has been unable to contact him due to a disconnected phone, and after contacting local law enforcement, a welfare check reveals that he is living at home without power, heat, or phone due to failing to pay the last three utility bills.

Discussion
Medical treatments, both with medication and other modalities, can have a significant impact on FDMC. The amnesia induced by ECT is most often transient but can have impairments that compound with those of the depression itself. Since the amnesia often recovers at 3 months [11, 12], it would be important to monitor patients closely in the post-procedure period until they have recovered. When patients do not have a ready proxy to monitor their finances, it may be important to assign DPOA prior to ECT or a case worker.

Example 3
A 92-year-old man arrives with his granddaughter. His wife of 64 years died 3 years ago, and she was the primary person managing the household finances. Most of their investments have been conservative, such as certificates of deposits or mutual funds. However, the granddaughter notes that recently he has been making increasingly risky investment choices, such as buying "stock" in an unlisted company, and sending large checks ($20,000 was the most recent one) to an overseas address. He does not appear to be forgetful and still can cook for himself and do basic laundry.

Discussion
In this final case, we see a patient with an isolated concern – risk-taking behavior – in the background of otherwise intact instrumental activities of daily living. While risk-taking behaviors may change with age, individuals in early stages of dementia may show a shift in decision-making toward being less risk-averse. Individuals with dementia may manifest this by shifting from a history of relatively conservative investment strategies to taking on more "high risk, high gain" products without truly understanding the consequences. Impairment in the ability to understand such risks or absorb the details of complex financial products puts such individuals at risk for exploitation. While this person's financial activities may raise concern for financial exploitation or fraud and practical consequences of poor investment choices, there should also be a concern that such changes in behavior may indicate underlying cognitive impairment, and testing to see if cognitive impairment exists would be recommended. In cases where assistance with financial decision-making is indicated, choosing the least restrictive option to help him manage his financial affairs appropriately should be considered.

Conclusion

Healthcare providers are often faced with ethical dilemmas involved in assessing a person's decision-making capacity. Impaired financial decision-making capacity, while less often recognized and evaluated, can have a significant impact on a person's health and well-being. Any signs of impaired FDMC (revealed by the patient or those around them) should lead to direct assessment of cognitive function as it can be one of the earliest signs of dementia. While neuropsychological testing is the most comprehensive assessment, shorter assessment tools that have tasks that test planning and calculation, such as the SLUMS test illustrated above, may be preferable as a starting point and may identify the areas of cognitive impairment that are directly affecting that individual's FDMC.

Acknowledgments The current author would like to acknowledge the efforts and work of the previous author of this chapter – Thomas Price, MD, Emory University School of Medicine, Division of General Medicine and Geriatrics, Atlanta, GA.

References

1. The next four decades: the older population in the United States: 2010 to 2050 [monograph online]. Washington, DC: US Census Bureau; 2010 [cited 2013 Nov 11]. Available from: http://www.census.gov/prod/2010pubs/p25-1138.pdf.
2. Vital and health statistics, National health interview study 2011. Washington, DC: US Department of Health and Human Services; Dec 2012.
3. Applebaum PS. Assessment of patient's competence to consent to treatment. N Engl J Med. 2007;357:1834–40.
4. Widera E, Steenpass V, Marson D, et al. Finances in the older patient with cognitive impairment. JAMA. 2011;305(7):698–706.
5. Valcour VG, Masaki KH, Curb JD, et al. The detection of dementia in the primary care setting. Arch Intern Med. 2000;160(19):2964–8.
6. Rule NO, Slepian ML, Ambady N. A memory advantage for untrustworthy faces. Cognition. 2012;125:207–18.
7. Dror IE, Katona M, Mungur K. Age differences in decision making: to take a risk or not? Gerontology. 1998;44:67–71.
8. Borson S, Scanlan J, Brush M, et al. The mini-cog: a cognitive "vital signs" measure for dementia screening in multi-lingual elderly. Int J Geriatr Psychiatry. 2000;15(11):1021–7.
9. Tariq SH, Tumosa N, Chibnall JT, et al. Comparison of the Saint Louis University mental status examination and the mini-mental state examination for detecting dementia and mild neurocognitive disorder – a pilot study. Am J Geriatr Psychiatry. 2006;14(11):900–10.
10. Feliciano L, Horning SM, Klebe KJ, et al. Utility of the SLUMS as a cognitive screening tool among a nonveterean sample of older adults. Am J Geriatr Psychiatry. 2012;21(7):623–30. https://doi.org/10.1016/j.jagp.2013.01.024.
11. Folstein MF, Folstein SE, McHugh PR. Mini-mental state. A practical method for grading the cognitive state of patients for the clinician. J Psychiatr Res. 1975;12(3):189–98.
12. Meeter M, Murre JMJ, Janssen SMJ, Birkenhager T, et al. Retrograde amnesia after electroconvulsive therapy: a temporary effect? J Affect Disord. 2011;132(1):216–22.

Chapter 8
Financial Exploitation: The Legal Perspective

Adam M. Fried, Franklin C. Malemud, and Page B. Ulrey

Introduction

The fight against financial exploitation of our elderly population requires a strong interrelation between the medical, financial, and legal systems to be effective. Before the courts can protect the elderly from financial exploitation and other abuses, persons having frontline access must first be able to recognize it. Unfortunately, exploitation can be difficult to identify for the simple reason that the transaction(s) at issue might appear to be the result of legitimate choice. Major transfers of an elder's assets occur for a wide variety of reasons ranging from love, affection, and generosity to exploitation and abuse. Somewhere in between is a blurred line over which a legitimate transaction ends and an exploitive one begins. This chapter, by case examples and through an explanation of the legal principles involved, seeks to arm the medical professional and others on the front lines with the tools necessary to identify patients at risk for exploitation, assist with intervention, and prevent their exploitation in the future.

A. M. Fried · F. C. Malemud (✉)
Reminger Co. LPA, Cleveland, OH, USA

Probate and Trust Litigation, Cleveland, OH, USA

P. B. Ulrey
King County Prosecutor's Office, Seattle, WA, USA

R. M. Factora (ed.), *Aging and Money*,
https://doi.org/10.1007/978-3-030-67565-3_8

Financial Exploitation: A Blurred Line

The 86-year-old Louise sat in her living room, papers and old mail cluttering the floor and furniture around her. Next to her were a lawyer and her ex-son-in-law, Paul, whom she had appointed to be her financial power of attorney. Paul convened the meeting to convince Louise of the benefit of selling the home in which she and her mother before her were raised. Louise had repeatedly told anyone who would listen that she wanted to die in her family home [1]. Paul said the problem was that if her care needs required her to be admitted into a nursing home, her home would need to be sold in order to pay for her care. Paul and an attorney he had contacted came to Louise with a solution: sell her home to Paul, he would lease the property back to her at no charge for the rest of her life, and she would have sufficient funds to pay for care. Believing that this was the right thing to do, Louise agreed and signed the documents. At the time she did this, she had been diagnosed with moderate dementia and had deferred all of her financial management to Paul. Within several months of the sale, Paul sent Louise to live with a caretaker whom she had never met before. Instead of using the money generated from the sale to allow Louise to remain in her home, Paul used the money to pay for updates to the property he now owned.

Louise is not alone. Consumers Digest estimates that there are five million victims of elder abuse, neglect, and exploitation every year [2]. The Government Accountability Office estimated that 14% of the population of those 65 years or older has been subject to some form of elder abuse [3]. MetLife Mature Market Survey estimated that the elder population is exploited out of $2.6 billion in assets annually [4]. While statistics as to the incidence of financial exploitation vary substantially, the consensus is that there is a "[l]arge reservoir of unreported and undetected cases of elder mistreatment about which very little is known" [5]. The problem of underreporting is exacerbated by the fact that "Victims of elder mistreatment infrequently seek help for the problem on their own; therefore, by the time the case has progressed to the point at which it is detected by a service agency, it is often very complex and difficult to treat" [6].

It is often similarly difficult to prove financial abuse when a case is presented to the court system. The legal complexities of these cases arise from two competing principles of American jurisprudence: the prized right of autonomy, privacy, and the freedom to gift versus the government's duty to protect those who are unable to protect themselves. Americans place tremendous value on privacy rights and the ability to do that which they please with their property. On the other hand, older adults who are financially exploited suffer tremendously painful consequences upon loss of their assets, including loss of the ability to pay for care, alienation from family, and even premature death [7]. Mickey Rooney, a famous American actor, explained the concept well when he testified before Congress that "What other people see as generosity may, in reality, be the exploitation, manipulation, and sadly, emotional blackmail of older, more vulnerable members of the American public" [8]. If an exploitative transaction between a vulnerable adult and the recipient can appear to be the result of generosity, then it corresponds that the ability to legally prove the transaction was instead the product of exploitation can be quite difficult.

The difficulty lies in the fact that an exploited person often expresses apparent consent and seems to support the transaction despite the fact that the transaction is based on manipulation, threats, deception, and other forms of exploitation. At least one commentator on this subject has described the phenomenon of the appearance of consent as "tacit consent" and has observed that "[F]inancial abuse is more likely to occur with the tacit acknowledgement and consent of the elder person…" [9]. This is a dangerous concept, because in the busy practices of lawyers and doctors who routinely assist the elderly, it is all too simple to accept the outward appearance of consent. As Louise's case demonstrates, a case of tacit consent, upon deeper investigation, is often revealed to be the product of actual exploitation.

After Louise was forced to move from her home, her case was brought to the attention of Adult Protective Services (APS) who intervened and sought the appointment of a guardian. The guardian conducted his investigation and filed suit to recover Louise's home and the expenditures Paul had made as her financial power of attorney. Paul defended the lawsuit by claiming that this transaction was the product of Louise's free choice. The attorney he had brought to the transaction testified that he was Louise's independent counsel and that she had consented to and supported the transaction. If the testimony of Louise's attorney was to be accepted, it could be said that Louise had tacitly consented to the transaction which led to her ultimate ouster from her home. However, the truth behind her apparent consent was that the transaction resulted from exploitive behavior that was only visible after an independent investigation into Louise's cognitive capacity, her relationship with Paul, the statements Paul made to her about the transaction, and Paul's handling of Louise's finances.

The court ruled on the side of the guardian, set aside the troublesome transaction, and restored Louise's property to her. The "consent," as the involved attorney described, turned out not to be consent at all. The court determined that Paul had downplayed Louise's cognitive decline and that the attorney had failed to ask pertinent questions or otherwise had ignored evidence of exploitation, partly because of his allegiance to Paul. Further, though Paul had represented to Louise that the transaction was designed to protect her ability to live in her home until death, it in fact enabled Paul to oust Louise from her home in a matter of months. Even the basis behind the transaction was misrepresented to Louise. She was informed that the home needed to be protected for Medicaid purposes in part because her finances had dwindled to such a state that she could not afford nursing services. In reality, Louise had sufficient resources to pay for such services; instead, Paul, as her power of attorney, used much of the money he paid for the property to "fix it up" for his own benefit. Louise's case was successfully pursued by APS in large part because she had been deemed incompetent,[1] which enabled the agency to pursue its investigation without her input. The harder cases to prevent and/or remedy are those that

[1] Many state laws use the word "incapacity" and "incapacitated" when referring to incompetence. Practitioners should refer to their own state laws in determining which word to use.

involve vulnerable older persons who, though susceptible to undue influence, are not, in a traditional view, incompetent. Such persons are often "strong-willed" yet easily manipulated by the exploiter, usually because the exploiter has gone to great lengths to cultivate the elder's trust. These vulnerable, yet competent, adults might see their independence as tied up in their relationship with the exploiter or might be too afraid of the ramifications should they resist. It is necessary to understand the manner in which vulnerable, yet competent, adults are exploited in order to devise the tools necessary to protect our elder population from exploitation.

The Concept of Undue Influence as a Mechanism to Exploit

At its very core, undue influence is the concept by which a perpetrator causes a victim to do that which they would not have done but for the act of improper influence. Put another way, a person uses power and control to exploit the elders' trust, dependency, and fear in order to obtain their "consent" to one or many financial transactions. While many financial decisions are the result of some influence, decisions must be "undue" or exploitive in order to constitute undue influence. Courts have found that undue influence can be accomplished in "a myriad of ways" [10] often described as illegitimate [11], excessive/inordinate [12], dominating [13], pressuring [14], forceful [15], constraining [16], and deceptive [17]. However, just because undue influence can be described does not mean that it can be spotted easily. Victims of undue influence are often isolated and living alone in their own homes. Undue influence is typically perpetrated in private and without the knowledge of the elder's family or friends.

Some of the red flags of undue influence that the legal system has identified include the following signs or symptoms of the elder:

- Loneliness or isolation
- Recent loss of a spouse, partner, or other strong social support
- Poor physical health
- Mild cognitive impairment
- Drug/alcohol dependence
- Decline in self-care, i.e., failure to take medications as prescribed, to attend appointments or to follow through with physician's advice
- Recent changes to decision-making authority, i.e., perpetrator is added to bank account or will, appointed as power of attorney, or takes over elder's bill-paying responsibilities
- Uncharacteristic and/or abrupt changes in long-standing relationship, business, medical, or financial structures
- Unpaid bills

The perpetrator's behaviors that might be symptomatic of undue influence are the following:

- Isolating the elder
- Alienating the elder from family, friends, or community
- Undermining the elder's confidence in his/her own abilities
- Lying to or manipulating the elder
- Playing on the elder's fear of losing his/her independence
- Showing excessive concern over spending on medical care for the elder's benefit
- Creating a siege mentality wherein the elder is unable to believe that others around them are acting in the elder's best interests
- Showing unduly controlling behavior toward the elder

Taken individually, these red flags might not be significant. But when a number of them are present, clinicians should be concerned that undue influence might be occurring.

As noted by a father/son team of psychiatrists:

> The modus operandi [of the perpetrator of undue influence] is to offer themselves as a savior, healer, advocate, or protector and, over time, cause the elder to sever relationships with friends, business associates, and family, thereby isolating the 'victim.' They instill paranoia and suspicion in the victim to increase his or her sense of helplessness and dependency on the perpetrator. When the victims have been adequately brainwashed into believing that no one else cares for them or that [their heirs] are either helpless to positively affect their situation or, worse, are plotting against them, the perpetrator makes his or her ongoing support and 'protection' contingent on receiving increased financial control or remuneration [18].

For these reasons, transactions that are the product of undue influence are often insidious and difficult to prevent. Professionals, including healthcare providers, lawyers, bankers, and other financial advisors, run the risk of being manipulated into believing that the transaction at issue is a product of the elder's free will. For example, in one case in which one of the authors was involved, a patient's daughter asked the patient's primary care physician, who was unaware of his patient's complete medical history, to write a letter assessing the patient's general capacity. He wrote the following:

> Mrs. Jane is a patient of mine. I have provided her general primary care for many years. I have been asked to write a statement regarding her general cognitive function. It is noted that the patient has suffered from intermittent delirium which has been treated episodically with complete resolution of symptoms. The patient does not demonstrate any obvious cognitive impairment and has been able to make decisions regarding her medical care.

At the time he wrote this letter, the doctor had not seen the patient for several months. The patient's daughter, acting as the patient's historian, was known to the doctor since she was a patient herself. It was the daughter who told the doctor the mother's delirium had resolved completely. However, the daughter failed to tell the doctor that the mother had also been treated elsewhere. Had the doctor inquired, medical records from other treatment providers would have revealed that she had been diagnosed with severe dementia and ongoing episodes of confusion. In the meantime, the daughter-historian greatly benefitted from the change to her mother's estate plan which a lawyer agreed to write because he had received the doctor's letter. By failing to independently evaluate his patient's condition, the doctor unwittingly became the exploiter's tool, and the doctor's credibility was diminished after his patient's true medical condition was revealed through other sources.

Another example of undue influence is the case of John Doe.[2] John was an elderly widower. His circle of support consisted of his three loving children. They spent time with him throughout the week, took him to doctors' appointments, and helped him pay bills because he was legally blind and could not read the bills or see well enough to write out the checks. John had a sharp mind, was strong-willed, and managed his own investments with the help of a trusted professional advisor.

All was well until John suffered a significant medical event and landed in the hospital. For a short time, he was delusional and the medical team wanted John to be discharged to a nursing facility for observation. John railed against that possibility and found two young "friends," Stacy and Jim, who were acquaintances of his but were strangers to his children. John was happy when his "friends" came to visit. They reminded John that he was his own person and that no one, including his children, could force him to move into a nursing home. Jim and Stacy told John that they would figure out a way to get him out of the hospital. To John, these "friends" offered an escape from the life of dependence that he perceived was being forced on him by his children.

While he was in the hospital, John's children became suspicious about Jim and Stacy when John asked the children to retrieve his checkbook from home. An otherwise frugal man, John wanted to write a check to his friends for $5000 because they were nice to him. A power struggle ensued. The "friends" hired an attorney, previously unknown to John, for the purpose of removing the children and appointing Jim and Stacy as John's powers of attorney for his healthcare and financial decisions. During the next several months, John, with the help of his friends, checked out of the hospital against medical advice, fired his long-time attorney, replaced his money manager, and added Jim and Stacy's names to many of his financial accounts.

In response, John's children obtained a "Statement of Expert Evaluation" from John's treating physician in which the doctor opined that John was incompetent and in need of a guardian.[3] John's children then initiated a legal proceeding to have a guardian appointed over their father.

[2] John Doe is a fictionalized name based on an actual case handled by one of the authors.

[3] The term "guardian" is defined by law and in some states is equivalent to "conservator." However, in other states, such as Ohio, a conservator is appointed for a competent adult at the request of the adult. To avoid confusion, the authors will refer to "guardian," and the practitioner should consult the laws of their particular state to determine the proper usage of the term.

In the guardianship trial that ensued, John Doe testified adamantly that his children were to blame because they had tried to take away his independence and force him to move into a nursing home and that he wanted Jim and Stacy to benefit. His new attorney testified that he fervently believed that John was acting of his own free will and volition. The psychologist retained by John and his friends testified that it was his opinion that John was competent and not in need of a guardian. Neither the psychologist nor the new lawyer was aware of the recent action that Jim and Stacy had taken with regard to John's finances. The clinicians who testified observed that John's beliefs about his children resulted from false information given him by Jim and Stacy. Other testimonies showed that the actions that Jim and Stacy had taken were against John's best interests from both a financial and medical perspective.

The Role of the Clinician

In all cases where unnatural transactions or unusual generosity is present, the observations of clinicians who are providing medical care to the elder are essential to the civil and criminal justice systems' ability to intervene. The observations, if recorded and properly detailed, can help a court or other adult advocate take necessary action to protect the elder and his or her assets. A clinician can do great service by reporting the exploitation early and by assisting investigators and lawyers as they attempt to gather the necessary information that is later presented in court to demonstrate exploitation. In most states, medical providers are mandatory reporters who must report evidence of abuse and exploitation to Adult Protective Services and/or law enforcement. Because of this obligation, and the fact that the practitioner might well end up being a witness in a subsequent legal proceeding, it is essential that they be detailed and careful in their note-taking. Because the caregiver might well be the perpetrator, the practitioner should make certain to talk to the patient alone. The clinician should go beyond basic, conclusory questioning of the older patient, i.e., are you afraid for your safety, and inquire into details of the elder's life. If the clinician becomes aware of any uncharacteristic events that have occurred with regard to the elder's legal or financial situation, he/she should inquire into the elder's thought process behind those events. The practitioner should make every effort to thoroughly document any signs of possible financial exploitation that he or she has observed. Further, the clinician should document any and all signs of dementia and/or other cognitive impairments that he or she observes. When such signs are present, a thorough assessment of the patient's cognitive impairment is of paramount importance. Such an assessment must include testing not only of the patient's memory but also of his or her executive function. The Mini-Mental Status Examination, which tests only for memory impairment, is on its own and extremely inadequate tool with which to assess impairment of financial capacity or rational judgment.

While state and federal privacy laws usually protect information contained within patient history, clinicians need to be aware that it is common for investigators and attorneys on these cases to obtain access to the elder's medical records through a search warrant, a subpoena, or a court order. Because medical records are created at the time the patient's symptoms are observed and by a person disinterested in the underlying dispute, these hold great weight in determining the outcome of a legal case.

The Legal System: A Focus on Victim or Perpetrator

The American justice system is composed of two parts: civil and criminal. Depending on the case, either or both of these justice system components can remedy financial exploitation. The criminal justice system begins its focus on the victim, but when that victim refuses assistance, one can step in to help only when it is demonstrated that the victim is incompetent and thus unable to help themselves.

The civil system generally involves litigation between parties seeking relief by way of recovering money to compensate for loss, ordering another to take or refrain from certain action, and/or for a declaration of rights as to a certain thing such as a bank account, interest in a trust, or other assets. The remedies sought in civil cases typically involve money or property and cannot result in incarceration. In cases involving incompetent adults, the civil system also has in place a process which allows the court to step in and protect the individual(s) and/or their assets through the guardianship process.[4] If successful, such a process removes the incompetent person from the decision-making process and puts in place a substitute decision-maker.

Once a case moves forward in the criminal justice system, the focus shifts to the perpetrator. Cases are filed in the criminal justice system by federal, state, or local prosecutors when it is determined that a person has committed a crime in the relevant jurisdiction. Criminal cases are considered to be crimes against the government and are not dependent on the victim to initiate. This section will focus on the dynamics of the two legal systems and the manner in which they can be used separately or in conjunction with each other to solve the difficult problem of exploitation.

Civil Justice and the Concept of Protection for the Elderly

As a general rule, the civil justice system can step in only to protect a person from being exploited if the exploitation is noticed and brought to the attention of the court.[5] However, the ability of the court actually to protect that individual relates to

[4] In some states, the term "guardian" or "guardianship" is referred to as a "conservator" or "conservatorship." As used herein, the authors are referring to the highest form of court control with a corresponding aspect of legal loss of decision-making.

[5] This chapter concentrates on the protection mechanisms available to prevent exploitation from occurring and not the process by which damage resulting to an heir who has been disinherited by the exercise of undue influence can be remedied by way of civil lawsuit. Therefore, the concept of post mortem lawsuits to set aside wills, trusts, and other transactions will not be discussed herein to any great degree.

the severity of the individual's susceptibility. For example, a person who is found to be incompetent is no longer legally capable to make decisions, and a guardian can be appointed who will then be able to remedy the exploitation by taking possession of his or her assets. On the other end of the spectrum, a court will not intervene to protect a competent person who wants to give his or her money away to a "bad" person for "bad" reasons. It is the in-between case, where exploitation is clear but where the individual who has not been determined incompetent is helpless to recognize or prevent the exploitation, which presents the most trouble for the civil courts. Ultimately, the medical and legal communities must answer the pinnacle question regarding the manner in which incompetence is diagnosed and proven.

Each state has the power to create its own legal definition for incompetence. Therefore, medical providers should consult the rules of their own jurisdictions before rendering opinions that their patients are incompetent. Ohio defines "incompetent" in a typical manner as "[A]ny person who is so mentally impaired as a result of a mental or physical illness or disability, or mental retardation, or as a result of chronic substance abuse, that the person is incapable of taking proper care of the person's self or property or fails to provide for the person's family or other persons for whom the person is charged by law to provide . . . ." Broken down, the legal definition of incompetent requires the following: (a) mental impairment; (b) caused by physical or mental disease, disability, or illness; (c) that is sufficient to; and (d) render that person incapable of taking proper care of their person or property.

Because the legal test of "incompetence" cannot be met without a medical opinion, the guardianship application process usually requires a physician, or some other acceptable medical personnel, to sign a certification that the individual over whom the application is filed (known as the prospective "ward") is incompetent and in need of a guardian. Additionally, a mandatory reporter – such as a physician – filing a report of suspected abuse or exploitation can trigger an Adult Protective Services' investigation and a subsequent application for guardianship. In some cases where exploitation is suspected, the court will order an independent medical evaluation if there is sufficient evidence to suggest the victim is impaired and/or that exploitation is in process. Once the application or petition is filed, the prospective ward is notified and afforded the right to defend against the claim that he or she is incompetent. Furthermore, clear and convincing evidence must be presented to prove that a prospective ward is incompetent. In the absence of clear and convincing evidence of incompetence, the application is denied, and the vulnerable adult will be free to continue his/her relationship with the exploiter.

Consider again the case of John Doe, who you will recall happily discharged his attorney and doctors and disowned his family believing that they were out to get him. He was well aware of the nature and extent of his assets. He managed his own finances but required assistance because he was blind and could not read his bills or write his own checks. There was a disagreement as to the extent of his impairments, with several treating physicians diagnosing him as suffering from mild dementia but an expert he hired diagnosed him with intermittent and resolved delirium and deemed him capable of making his own decisions. If one were only to consider his mental acuity, then it would be difficult to say that he was incompetent and in need of a guardian. But, if his beliefs about his children were delusional, arising from manipulation by his exploiters, then was he incapable of taking care of his own person or property? Further, if his inability to recognize the inherent self-interest in the advances of his new "friends" resulted from his medical condition, then is an opinion of incompetence medically sound? There is some support, though limited, in the medical literature to suggest that a person may be incompetent because of the influence of third parties against whom that person is unable to protect [19].

The Role of the Medical Profession in the Civil Context

The medical profession plays a unique and critical role in the concept of protecting against the exploitation of the elderly in guardianship cases because the determination of incompetence is both a medical and a legal determination. In essence, the treating physician or a medical expert will assess the elder's competency, and the civil legal system will decide if the legal test of incompetence has been met based upon the medical and factual evidence. In that sense, the observations of the physician as to the manner in which the patient's thought process is affected by the conduct of third persons should be considered.

For example, in a case of a son exploiting his physically dependent elderly mother, the court found useful a patient medical history from treating doctors and from an assisted living facility. The mother had named her son as her power of attorney to assist her with her finances when she moved into an assisted living facility [20]. The son visited his mother often and assumed the handling of her financial affairs. The daughter also visited her mother regularly and was equal beneficiary of her mother's will, demonstrating her intent to treat her children equally. The mother never changed her will. Without advising the daughter, the son brought a form to his mother designating him as the sole beneficiary of her annuities and directing gifts to the son and his family. After the mother died, the daughter sued her brother in probate court regarding their mother's assets.

The court put weight in a geriatric psychiatrist's expert opinion, which contained an examination of the elder's medical records going back 6 years prior to the questioned exploitation. The detailed medical records established a base line with preexisting depression and anxiety problems that progressed into Alzheimer's-type dementia syndrome coupled with behavior problems, anxiousness, agitation, and paranoia. In relying on a detailed patient history, the geriatric psychiatrist opined that what began as a mild cognitive decline with short-term memory issues progressed into the patient being "very confused" with a substantial decline in her mental faculties. The psychiatrist further noted that medical personnel had documented "her short-term memory impairment and orientation problems," delusional stories, and her poor recollection and had regularly conducted regular Mini-Mental Status Examinations. The written patient history permitted the psychiatrist to present an expert opinion that supported the court's ruling that the patient was unable to manage her "own affairs and legally unable to give her property to anyone or any institution," resulting in undoing the financial exploitation. Without such a detailed patient history, the geriatric psychiatrist might not have been effective in being able to chart the decedent's progress toward incapacity.

In a similar case, daughters sought to invalidate a 1994 last will and testament on the grounds that their mother lacked the capacity to sign the document [21]. The will was presented at a time when the mother had questioned the capacity and persons close to her were exploiting her. The court was presented with medical records from 1993 forward showing that the decedent suffered from dementia, a progressive deterioration of intellectual functioning, and a delusion as to family history that was secondary to the decedent's demented condition. A treating doctor's report stated that during a 2-year period, two standardized psychological tests administered to the exploited and a clinical interview provided the following: "Mental Status evaluation and intellectual assessment [conducted in 1993] indicated [she was] experiencing Dementia-Mild type." A jury relied upon this evidence to conclude that the mother was incompetent, invalidate the last will and testament, and rectify the exploitation.

The Criminal Justice System at Work

In understanding the role of the criminal justice system in these cases, it is important to be aware of the fact that criminal prosecution of financial exploitation of the elderly is a fairly new phenomenon. Like domestic violence and child abuse, elder financial exploitation historically has been perceived to be a private matter or, at best, one for the civil court system. Only recently has it begun to be treated as a crime with any degree of consistency. Still, the progress of the criminal justice system in pursuing these cases is painfully slow. Only a small percentage of police officers, detectives, prosecutors, and 911 dispatchers are trained on how to recognize and properly respond to these cases. Without that training, reports of elder financial exploitation are often not investigated by the police. Even if a case is investigated, prosecutors do not often file charges. The reason training is necessary for these professionals is because these cases are almost always complicated, requiring knowledge of concepts such as powers of attorney, guardianships, conservatorships, dementia, capacity, and competency. Further, they require access to experts who can analyze financial documents, conduct capacity evaluations, and assist in the interpretation of medical records. Compounding all of this is the fact that these cases are often reported to the police long after the exploitation has occurred, creating significant proof problems for the prosecution, should the case gets that far. This being said, the situation is not all bad. Awareness of elder financial exploitation by the criminal justice system is increasing. Some jurisdictions now have specialized elder-abuse detectives and prosecutors, resulting in faster and more effective investigations and more prosecutions of these crimes.

This increased awareness on the part of the criminal justice system, combined with the general increase in reporting of these crimes, inevitably will result in increased requests for information and assistance from the medical field. In order that practitioners understand the nature of these requests and the impacts on a prosecution, it is important that they understand the process by which a criminal case is investigated and prosecuted.

When a 911 call is made or law enforcement receives a report from APS, patrol officers should respond, conduct an initial investigation, and, if further investigation is required, forward the case to a detective.[6] Detectives investigate financial cases by executing search warrants for the victim's and suspect's financial records and, often, for the victim's medical records. They interview the victim, the suspect, and other potential witnesses. They might also arrange for a competency evaluation of the victim. At the conclusion of their investigation, if the evidence is sufficient, detectives forward the case to the prosecutor's office for the filing of criminal charges. In more complex cases, prosecutors often work with detectives as the investigation progresses, advising them on what additional evidence is needed and occasionally participating in witness interviews. Once law enforcement refers a case, prosecutors review it and determine whether sufficient evidence exists to file charges. After charges are filed, prosecutors appear at the various hearings on the case, negotiate a possible resolution, and, if the defendant chooses to go to trial rather than plead guilty, try the case. In a criminal trial, it is the prosecutor's burden to prove the case to a jury beyond a reasonable doubt. The defendant need not put on any evidence, present any witnesses, or testify him or herself. Conviction of the offender can result in the issuance of no-contact orders, court-ordered treatment, jail or prison time for the offender, and, occasionally, return of some or all of the victim's stolen assets through an order of restitution.

In the vast majority of elder financial cases that end up before the criminal justice system, the perpetrator claims that the elder consented to the financial transactions. Thus, a key part of the investigation of the case involves determining whether the elder had the capacity to consent to the transactions at the time these occurred. An essential means of establishing the degree of the elder's impairment at the time of the incident is through the elder's medical records. If created by a conscientious healthcare provider, those records contain essential information about the elder's cognitive status during the time of the transactions, including signs and symptoms of impairment, assessments, diagnoses, and prescribed medications. Because the healthcare provider might be one of the few people who is observing and monitoring the elder during the time of the exploitation, he or she likely is to be an essential witness in the case against the exploiter.

---

[6] In smaller jurisdictions, these patrol officers may be tasked with the job of conducting the additional investigation themselves.

The Case of L.S.: The Need for Multidisciplinary Awareness and Interaction to Protect the Vulnerable from Devastating Loss

The case of L.S. is an example of the need for awareness across disciplines of exploitation signs and for a strategic approach to implement protections in a timely manner. In this case, the criminal justice system, through the actions of dedicated police, investigators, and prosecutors, eventually brought to justice an opportunistic predator and sent her to prison for the exploitation of her elderly, cognitively impaired victim. However, despite the involvement of friends, family, medical professionals, and the police, no protection was offered to the victim until long after the damage was done and until the victim himself agreed to tell his story. This example will be used to demonstrate the process by which the exploitation occurred and to discuss what strategies could have been employed by healthcare providers and other professionals to prevent the abuse in its earlier stages.

L.S. was mildly developmentally delayed, and prior to the untimely and tragic death of his wife of 34 years, he relied on her to handle all of the family's finances. The couple owned their home and had life insurance policies, health insurance, and very little debt. Several years before the exploitation began, a drunk driver struck and killed L.S.'s wife. In an instant, L.S. had lost his best friend, social support, partner, and protector.

After his wife's death, L.S., then 65 years old, began to frequent a bar near his house. There, he met the 43-year-old Lisa O'Neill. O'Neill had a long-term boyfriend, sporadic employment, and a great deal of debt. On the night they met, L.S. told O'Neill about his wife's death, as well as the fact that he was expecting a significant payoff from her life insurance policy. After drinking together for several hours, O'Neill convinced L.S. to come home with her. L.S. agreed and, within a couple of weeks, had moved into O'Neill's basement. Within a month, on the assumption that O'Neill would marry him, L.S. gave O'Neill $23,000 to pay off debt. Thus began a pattern of L.S. giving O'Neill substantial sums of money.

L.S. had three adult children. Several weeks after her father had suddenly moved out of his home, his daughter, Beverly, looked at L.S.'s bank statements. She noticed large, frequent withdrawals that were completely uncharacteristic of her father's spending patterns. Eventually, when her father would not return her phone calls, she called his bank and the police. The bank informed her that because her father appeared to have the capacity, there was nothing it could do. The police said virtually the same thing. Neither could provide any assistance to her. Soon thereafter, O'Neill, with L.S.'s apparent consent, moved his financial accounts to new institutions, took complete control over those accounts, and systematically began to drain him of all of his assets.

Early in the time he was living with O'Neill, L.S. suffered a stroke while at work and was hospitalized. As a result of the stroke, his speech was significantly impaired, and his left side was weakened. O'Neill did not visit him or contact him while he was at the hospital. Eventually, he was discharged back to his own home and his son's care. The discharge instructions included referrals for speech and physical therapy, medications, and follow-up visits. A short time after his discharge, L.S. went back to work. On his first day back, O'Neill drove to his workplace, approached him, and convinced him to move back in with her, promising that she would take care of him. L.S. stopped taking the medications that had been prescribed after his stroke, stopped attending his physical and speech therapy, and never returned to his treating physician for follow-up visits. The care promised to L.S. was not provided by O'Neill.

O'Neill's increasing emotional and sometimes physical abuse of L.S. marked the following months. She began to call him names like "moron," "faggot," and "leprechaun." When they went out with her friends, L.S. reported, "[she told me] not to say nothing to nobody else. Don't talk. Don't talk at all…I couldn't talk good anyways, so she told me to be quiet." When she became frustrated with L.S., O'Neill began to hit him or shove him. Over time, she turned L.S. against his children, convincing him they were after his money and that she was his protector.

A number of months after she obtained control of L.S.'s financial accounts, O'Neill stopped paying his bills. Eventually, foreclosure proceedings began on his home. O'Neill returned L.S.'s truck to the dealer from whom he had purchased it, telling L.S. he could no longer afford his truck payments. L.S.'s cell phone service was eventually cut off, leaving him without a means of communicating with anyone besides O'Neill and the people with whom she socialized.

By the summer of 2008, L.S. had lost his home, his truck, and most of his possessions. His relationships with his family and friends were estranged. He had nothing left. On a morning in July, L.S. woke up early, packed his things, and walked out O'Neill's front door and to the home of a friend several miles away. He told her his story, and she in turn called his children. His daughter Beverly arrived and promptly took her father to the local police department to make a report.

After a lengthy investigation, criminal charges were filed against Lisa O'Neill for the financial exploitation and abuse she inflicted on L.S. At trial, a geriatric psychiatrist testified that because of his developmental disability and vascular dementia, L.S. lacked financial capacity and was vulnerable to undue influence. Lisa O'Neill was found guilty of multiple counts of theft and sentenced to 62 months in prison.

By the time the system finally intervened on L.S.'s behalf, all of his assets were gone because O'Neill had spent all of L.S.'s money. Although the criminal court ordered O'Neill to pay restitution to L.S., L.S will be lucky if he receives even $25/month in restitution payments.

The systemic failures in this case were many. When L.S.'s daughter called the police and the bank, neither reported the matter to Adult Protective Services.[7] When

[7] In Washington, the state in which this crime occurred, law enforcement is a mandatory reporter of vulnerable adult abuse and exploitation. Banks are permissive reporters.

L.S. failed to follow through on his discharge instructions from the hospital, none of his medical providers reported his absence to APS. Had any of those professionals called APS, L.S. would have been contacted. If L.S. had a proper capacity assessment, a guardianship petition could have been filed. Criminal charges also could have been filed, and a no-contact or protection order obtained. All of these civil and criminal responses could have saved some portion of L.S.'s assets and significantly improved his quality of life.

Although what constitutes a crime of elder financial exploitation varies by state, virtually all states criminalize the taking of a senior's assets in the following situations:

- Perpetrator has a fiduciary relationship to the elder, i.e., is his or her power of attorney, guardian, conservator attorney, accountant, or bill payer, and uses the elder's assets for his or her own, rather than for the elder's benefit.
- Perpetrator obtains the elder's assets by deceiving the elder.
- Perpetrator takes the senior's assets without the senior's knowledge.
- Perpetrator obtains the senior's assets without the true consent of the elder (through undue influence, manipulation, or due to the senior's incapacity).

Despite the fact that these situations constitute a crime, whether the criminal justice system of a particular jurisdiction will treat these as such depends on the level of awareness and the training that has been conducted there, and on whether sufficient evidence, including documentation of the elder's cognitive status at the time of the exploitation, exists.

Recommendations and Conclusions

There can be little doubt that financial exploitation of your elderly patients is occurring and statistics show that it is occurring at an increasingly frequent rate. The first step to protecting your patients from harm is to understand and document their vulnerability to exploitation. Such documentation must start with an accurate diagnosis of the underlying condition(s) that make(s) the patient vulnerable and be followed by a thorough assessment of the patient's capacity to make particular decisions. As part of this assessment, clinicians must evaluate the patient's executive function, in addition to his or her memory. The healthcare professional needs to pay attention to signs of abuse or exploitation which, standing alone, might seem unimportant but, when viewed as a whole, might warrant a report. Because of the direct impact on the health, well-being, and longevity of your older patients, it is essential that exploitation and abuse be considered as a differential diagnosis.

To the same extent, recordkeeping needs to be clear and detailed so that a forensic review of the record accurately will reveal the circumstances that existed at the time of exploitation. The histories patients provide are incredibly important and also should be thoroughly documented. However, often the caregiver provides the patient history, alone or in conjunction with the patient. The practitioner should be careful to assign the actual provider of the history in the record, as evidence of a perpetrator's wrongdoing might be contained in the inaccurate history that he or she provides. In the same vein, concerning statements or behaviors of the perpetrator should also be documented.

Additionally, good recordkeeping aids the medical provider, especially if that provider is called as a witness in a civil or criminal proceeding related to the exploitation. In many of these cases, legal proceedings may not take place until years after the exploitation occurred. As a witness on the case, the provider will be entitled to rely on notes while testifying. With the accumulation of several years and thousands of patient visits between the practitioner and to what is being testified, the notes may be the only aid that may be relied upon to assist the practitioner in remembering what occurred.

While any exploitation from which the practitioner's patient is suffering likely will occur outside of their presence, the medical practitioner may be in a unique position to view the dynamics between the elder and his or her exploiter. Any red flags observed should cause lead to an inquiry into those dynamics to obtain more information about the patient's social and financial situation and cognitive status. Similarly, a patient believed to have sufficient means to obtain proper care but appears to be self-neglecting or is refusing treatment for alleged financial reasons should be questioned thoroughly about his or her home life and financial situation and assessed for cognitive impairment. Generally speaking, if at any point in the care of a patient a concern develops regarding his or her cognitive abilities, noting in detail the basis for concern and thoroughly testing that patient's cognitive function are essential. The practitioner's documentation of observations and the information obtained during examinations of such a patient might be critical factors in a subsequent criminal or civil proceeding involving this patient.

Finally, when there is suspicion that a patient is being abused or exploited, it should be reported. It is not up to the medical provider to determine whether abuse or exploitation is actually occurring. It is merely up to the provider to relay these concerns to the agencies that are responsible for that investigation. This report may be the very first information the system receives that this individual patient is being abused or exploited. This initial report may result in a civil or criminal intervention that could save that patient's assets and, ultimately, his or her life.

References

1. Thompson v. Radis. Cuyahoga County Probate Court Case # 2007 ADV 129205.
2. Wasik JF. The fleecing of America's elderly. Consum Dig. 2000;(5):78–9.
3. Report to the Chairman, Special Committee on Aging, U.S. Senate. Stronger Federal leadership could enhance national response to elder abuse. GAO-11-208. 2011. https://www.gao.gov/new.items/d11208.pdf
4. The MetLife Mature Market Institute et al., "Broken Trust: Elders, Family, and Finances – A Study on Elder Financial Abuse Prevention," 2009. https://www.gao.gov/new.items/d11208.pdf

5. Panel to Review Risk and Prevalence of Elder Abuse and Neglect. Elder mistreatment: abuse, neglect, and exploitation in an aging America. Washington, D.C.: The National Academies Press; 2003. p. 22.
6. Elder Mistreatment at p. 88.
7. Lachs MS, Willams C, O'Brien S, Pillemer K, Charlson ME. The mortality of elder mistreatment. JAMA. 1998;280:428–32.
8. Senate Special Committee on Aging. Testimony of Mickey Rooney. 2011.
9. Elder Mistreatment at p. 382.
10. In re Succession of Lounsberry. 824 So.2d 409, 412. 2002.
11. Looney v. Estate of Wade. 310 Ark. 708, 711. 1992.
12. In re Will Testament of Walls. 2009 Del. Ch. LEXIS 222, *21. 2009.
13. King v. MacDonald. 90 Idaho 272, 279. 1965.
14. In reWilley's Estate. 9 Mich. App. 245, 254-55. 1967.
15. Hamilton v. Steininger. 350 Mo. 698, 713. 1943.
16. Matter of Robinson's Estate. 231 Kan. 300, 306. 1982.
17. De Nieff v. Howell. 138 Ga. 248, 204. 1912.
18. RCW H, RCW H, Chapman MJ. Exploitation of the elderly: undue influence as a form of elder abuse. Clin Geriatr. 2005;13(2):30–1.
19. Spar JE, Hankin M, Stodden AB. Assessing mental capacity and susceptibility to undue influence. Behav Sci Law. 1995;13:391–403.
20. Schiavoni v. Roy. 9th Dist. No. 11CA0108-M, 2012-Ohio-4435, ¶¶ 2-3.
21. Bodenbender v. Long. 3d Dist. No. 4-95-11, 1996 Ohio App. LEXIS 1718, **11-14.

Chapter 9
Perspectives from Financial Institutions

Celiza P. Bragança and Lisa J. Bleier

Financial institutions, including banks, brokerage firms, and investment advisers, are working with elder advocates, regulators, and law enforcement to develop effective means to prevent exploitation of investors. This is of critical importance for a number of reasons. One is that persons age 65 and older have much greater wealth than their younger counterparts [1]. Median net worth of individuals in this age group averages around $271,162, as compared to $61,146 for people aged 35–44 [1]. This difference makes older individuals an attractive target for scammers. Scammers target older individuals for the same reason that Willie Sutton robbed banks – "because that's where the money is."

These institutions are also concerned about elder financial exploitation because of the incidence of cognitive impairment among this age group. In addition to the normal age-related decline in cognitive abilities, a significant number of people over 75 years of age have either mild cognitive impairment (MCI) or dementia (Petersen, NEJM, 2011). Despite the "mild" term used in mild cognitive impairment, this condition's impact on the individual's ability to make financial decisions is anything but mild. Persons with MCI make four times more financial decision-making errors compared to persons without MCI. Because those persons taking advantage of these at-risk elders are often family members, friends, or caregivers of their victim, victims often fail to report these incidents. A New York State Adult Protective Services (APS) study found that 67% of verified cases of financial exploitation were committed by family members – and only an estimated 1 in 44 cases are ever reported to the authorities. These victims can lose their entire life savings to these "bad actors," leaving them unable to maintain their independence or pay for their own healthcare,

C. P. Bragança (✉)
Bragança Law LLC, Skokie, IL, USA
e-mail: Lisa@SECDefenseAttorney.com

L. J. Bleier
SIFMA, Washington, DC, USA
e-mail: lbleier@sifma.org

R. M. Factora (ed.), *Aging and Money*,
https://doi.org/10.1007/978-3-030-67565-3_9

not to mention the added emotional stress, significant physical health impacts, and – often – the loss of important relationships.

There are numerous ways that older persons can be financially exploited. A great deal of the exploitation is by persons known and trusted by elders through abuse of powers of attorney, undue influence, and affinity fraud [2]. Undue influence is a legal doctrine that can apply when someone uses excessive persuasion to influence another person, particularly when the influenced person's capacity is limited. Affinity frauds exploit the trust that members of a group like a religious or ethnic community have in their fellow members. Exploitation of older persons by strangers often is by telephone. In those calls, fraudsters seek to take advantage of them through grandchildren scams (caller pretends to be a grandchild who needs money sent immediately), technical support scams (caller convinces the person to give them access to a computer or other electronic devices), imposter scams (caller claims to be someone whom the older person would help by sending money), charity scams (caller claims to be raising money for a charitable cause but is not), and identity theft (caller obtains personal identifiable information of older person to open and use credit card accounts, divert tax refunds, make purchases, etc.) [2].

Financial institutions have an opportunity to be a first line of defense against fraud and financial exploitation. All individuals who remain independent in the community need to access their money to pay for the basics of living. They do so by writing checks; withdrawing funds from bank accounts, investment advisory accounts, or brokerage accounts; and using credit cards. As a result, individuals are interacting with the financial services sector constantly. This gives "bad actors" many opportunities to access and obtain an older person's financial assets. But, as the Consumer Financial Protection Bureau (CFPB) notes, "banks and credit unions are uniquely positioned to detect that an older account holder has been targeted or victimized, and to take action" [3].

"Red flags" suggesting suspicious activity indicating potential elder financial exploitation may be recognized by financial institutions. Specific procedures have been developed and may be implemented when there is awareness of the presence of these red flags. In some cases, the response to such a red flag is to contact family, friends, or others in the customer's life circle. Here is an example of a case with a potential red flag:

> An 82-year-old customer, Deborah, lives in an assisted living facility and communicates regularly with her financial advisor. One day, Deborah calls the advisor and asks him to wire a large sum of money, explaining that she is buying a house in Costa Rica. The concerned financial advisor asks if Deborah has ever been to Costa Rica. Deborah says no, she just wanted to buy the home.

The employee of this financial institution has an opportunity to take action before monies are wired out from the funds of the customer's account. In this case, the financial advisor contacted the firm's lawyers who advised him to ask Deborah for the name of the attorney handling the purchase and the address of the property she is going to purchase in Costa Rica. Although Deborah calls her financial advisor daily asking for the funds transfer, she is not able to provide the name of the attorney or the address of the house she wants to buy. The financial advisor's manager calls Deborah, and ultimately Deborah tells him that she lied about the house and wants the money because she has won a sweepstakes lottery. The financial institution then contacted the director of the assisted living facility to alert them to this potential scam. The director, who overheard Deborah talking on the phone about winning a lottery, was able to work together with the financial institution to explain the scam to Deborah. The assisted living facility then helped Deborah change her phone number to stop the calls and held a seminar for its residents to educate them on scams and other elder financial exploitation issues.

This cascade of events and interventions all began with Deborah asking for a large wire from her investment account and concluded with a financial advisor, who knew to ask more questions, making the communications necessary to stop the transaction and educate the person who was targeted to be victimized (Deborah) and then facilitating changes in Deborah's contact information to prevent future scammers from contacting her again. This is an ideal situation where the employees of the institution responsible for Deborah's finances were concerned about the circumstances regarding her potential financial transaction and worked with their client and her residence to help clarify the rationale for her decision to avoid a potentially catastrophic decision. Financial institutions are training financial advisors and other personnel to take action when they become aware of these kinds of red flags.

Identifying Cognitive Decline Through Financial Interactions

As clients age, the threat of financial exploitation or cognitive decline grows exponentially, and financial institutions that become aware of the signs of cognitive decline or exploitation are able to ask more questions. Certain signs might be noticed by a financial advisor during interactions with a customer. While these signs are not specific indicators that fraud or exploitation is going to take place, they should compel the involved institution or agent to proceed with some heightened awareness as there may be a higher risk of these events happening to this individual. Signs of possible cognitive decline or exploitation include the following:

- Client is accompanied by a caregiver or family member who will not allow the client to speak without them being present.
- Client repeatedly calls seeking the same information.
- Client has atypical or unexplained withdrawals, wire transfers, debit transaction, or other changes in financial habits.
- Client abruptly changes their will, trusts, powers of attorney, or beneficiaries of their accounts.
- Client suddenly changes their investment style or begins trading excessively in high-risk instruments or has excessive outflows or trading losses.

Training personnel to identify red flags indicating possible elder financial exploitation has been a goal for many financial institutions [4]. For those financial institution that may only see a client for a brief snippet of time, these signs could very well have an innocuous explanation, but it is important for that institution to check to see what that explanation is and decide at that time whether or not additional inquiries and/or interventions are necessary to protect that client's assets.

What Can Financial Institutions Do and Not Do?

Financial institutions are regulated by numerous entities to protect the security and confidentiality of personal information of their customers. These laws and regulations can limit what financial institutions can do to respond to suspected elder financial exploitation. The primary law governing this space is the Gramm-Leach-Bliley Act which prevents financial institutions from disclosing nonpublic information about consumers [5]. There are few exceptions in the law, but many advocates have worked together to allow for the sharing of certain information relating to financial exploitation.

For years financial institutions have been working with legislators, regulators, and law enforcement to work on ways that they can report, as well as combat and mitigate, elder financial exploitation. Investment and brokerage firms, which are regulated by the US Securities and Exchange Commission at the federal level, state securities regulators, and self-regulatory organizations like FINRA (Financial Industry Regulatory Authority), recognize they have an important role to play in preventing and detecting elder financial exploitation. Firms and securities industry trade associations like SIFMA (Securities Industry and Financial Markets Association) have been working with regulators and legislators to make it legal for them to report suspected elder financial exploitation to Adult Protective Services (APS) and other government agencies.

In 2013, a group of federal regulators issued joint guidance regarding how the Gramm-Leach-Bliley Act [6] (which requires financial institutions to ensure the security and confidentiality of customer personal information) might be unduly limiting the reporting of suspected financial exploitation of older adults [7]. The guidance clarifies that reporting suspected financial exploitation of older adults to appropriate local, state, or federal enforcement agencies does not, in general, violate the privacy provisions of the Gramm-Leach-Bliley Act [8]. Some questions remained with regard to sharing of this type of information with nonenforcement agencies. As a result, in 2018 Congress enacted the Senior Safe Act to make it clear that banks and brokerage firms are permitted to share information relating to potential exploitation with APS and similar organizations without violating the Gramm-Leach-Bliley Act.

The Senior Safe Act allows financial institutions working with APS and similar agencies to disclose information that is required to be kept private under the Gramm-Leach-Bliley Act. Those institutions and financial services professionals are not liable for reporting suspected elder financial exploitation to these agencies as long as the financial professionals have been properly trained. Over time, more financial institutions have developed and implemented training that permits them to report suspected elder financial exploitation. Recently, APS organizations in cooperation with SIFMA, FINRA, and NASAA (North American Securities Administrators Association) developed and released guidelines for APS to work with financial institutions to respond to suspected elder financial exploitation [9].

In addition to reporting suspected elder financial exploitation, financial institutions may be able to prevent financial losses by delaying carrying out a customer's request that funds be paid out of an account to prevent a scam or fraud from taking place. However, doing so may violate the law [10].

In the last few years, a substantial number of states have enacted legislation based upon the State of Washington's law which was enacted in 2011 [11]. This law generally grants financial institutions and their employees' immunity for taking proactive steps to delay disbursements and report suspected elder financial exploitation to the appropriate authorities. Since then, the following states have enacted laws and/or regulations based upon this first law: Alabama, Alaska, Arizona, Arkansas, California, Colorado, Delaware, Indiana, Kentucky, Louisiana, Maine, Maryland, Minnesota, Mississippi, Montana, New Hampshire, New Mexico, North Dakota, Oregon, Tennessee, Texas, Utah, Vermont, and Virginia [12].

To encourage financial institutions to report financial exploitation, the Department of the Treasury's Financial Crimes Enforcement Network (FinCEN) added a box for "elder financial exploitation" on the Suspicious Activity Report (SAR) form that financial institutions are required to submit. An advisory issued in February 2011 provides a listing of signs of abuse that financial institutions might see [13]. Those signs of abuse include the following:

- Changes in appearance or personal hygiene
- Forgetfulness, memory lapses
- Fearfulness, distressed or submissive behavior
- Disorganized or disoriented behavior
- Change from previous personality and behavior

This data is used by the Department of Justice (DOJ) and others to analyze elder financial exploitation [14]. It is worth noting, however, that SARs are used for preventing money laundering and various federal and international crimes. The addition of the box with regard to financial exploitation assists only with tracking abuse and not with addressing an individual case.

Who Are the Relevant Federal and State Regulators?

There are a number of federal regulators who educate and combat elder financial exploitation. On the criminal side, the primary federal agency is the US Department of Justice. The DOJ includes the FBI and US Attorney's Offices throughout the country. Civil investigations and enforcement actions as well as rulemaking are covered by a number of federal agencies. The Securities and Exchange Commission (SEC) focuses on brokerage firms and investment advisory firms. The Consumer Financial Protection Bureau (CFPB) focuses on banks, lenders, and financial institutions, other than securities and investment firms. The CFPB publishes alerts and educational material concerning elder financial exploitation [15]. The Federal Trade Commission (FTC) has broad jurisdiction to protect consumers. The FTC covers some of the same bank, lender, and financial institution activity as the CFPB, but not the brokerage and investment activities covered by the SEC. The FTC also publishes information to educate and protect older consumers [16].

Most states have their own securities regulatory agency tasked with protecting investors, including elders, in their state. In addition, state attorneys general may investigate and bring actions for elder financial exploitation. Insurance products like equity-indexed annuities (also called fixed indexed annuities) are generally the responsibility of state insurance commissioners.

What Are Federal and State Regulators Doing?

The US Department of Justice is responsible for criminal prosecution of elder financial exploitation at the federal level. In 2017, Congress passed the Elder Abuse Prevention and Prosecution Act which required the DOJ to identify one federal prosecutor in each federal judicial district to investigate and prosecute elder financial exploitation. This law is intended to increase training for federal investigators and prosecutors, to equip each judicial district with prosecutors having expertise with elder exploitation cases, and overall to strengthen the ability of our justice system to respond when elder exploitation is identified, including when financial institutions report suspected financial exploitation. The DOJ has coordinated several "sweeps" of elder fraud cases and dedicated an entire issue of its *Journal of Federal Law and Practice* to elder financial exploitation [17]. The DOJ collects and reports on its actions to combat elder financial exploitation on its website [18]. States are also prosecuting more elder financial exploitation cases.

The SEC is active in combating elder financial exploitation through education and outreach and its examination program. The SEC Office of the Investor Advocate issued two white papers on elder financial exploitation: *Elder Financial Exploitation: Why it is a concern, what regulators are doing about it, and looking ahead* [19] and *How the SEC Works to Protect Senior Investors* [20]. In these white papers, the SEC details the work it has done and continues to do to balance the privacy and right of older investors to make their own financial decisions with the need to protect older investors from financial exploitation. The SEC has also published an investor bulletin entitled *Help for Adult Protective Services (APS) Workers Encountering Senior Investor Fraud* [21] to assist APS personnel in responding to signs of elder investment fraud.

For years, the SEC has made protecting senior retail investors one of its highest priorities in conducting its examination program. In 2015, the SEC and FINRA issued a joint report of their observations from examinations they conducted of broker-dealers and investment advisers [22]. They noted that brokerage firm employees should be trained on what steps to take to report signs of diminished capacity or elder financial abuse (*Id.* at 8.) The regulators noted that firms should establish strict guidelines to ensure that senior investors' holdings are not overconcentrated in certain products and engage in heightened supervision of investments by seniors in certain types of securities (*Id.* at 20, 29.)

The SEC and FINRA continue to make financial exploitation of older customers a priority in conducting their examinations [23]. In particular, the SEC and FINRA focus on the supervisory policies and procedures that firms have to protect senior investors:

> Protection of senior investors, as well as investors who are retired or approaching retirement, remains a top priority for FINRA and we will continue to focus on how firms are protecting such persons from fraud, sales practice abuses and financial exploitation. FINRA will assess firms' supervision of accounts where registered representatives serve in a fiduciary capacity, including holding a power of attorney, acting as a trustee or co-trustee, or having some type of beneficiary relationship with a non-familial customer account. In particular, we are concerned about registered representatives using their role as a fiduciary to take control of trusts or other assets and direct funds to themselves. FINRA will assess the supervisory systems firms employ to place heightened scrutiny over such accounts.

In the FINRA 2019 Annual Risk Monitoring and Examination Priorities Letter, the SEC staff note that policies and procedures concerning diminished capacity of customers should provide information about how to recognize the signs of diminished capacity and specific actions a person should take in such cases (SEC 2019 Examination Priorities, at 4). Red flags that could raise concerns include:

- Client informs you of a new "sweetheart."
- Client sounds "coached" over the phone.
- Client is dependent on another for care.
- Client repeatedly seeks the same information.
- Change in client's behavior noted.
- Abrupt changes to a client's will, trust, or powers of attorney are made.

In February 2018, FINRA enacted Rules 2165 and 4512. These rules have been helpful tools for financial advisers trying to protect investors from financial exploitation. Under new Rule 2165, a firm can delay an older customer's request for disbursement if the firm has a good faith belief that elder financial exploitation is taking place. This is a powerful tool that gives firms a pause to contact a client's friends and family members – and the appropriate authorities – *before* funds are transferred out of the client's account. Where the suspected exploiter is a family member, the pause gives firms the opportunity to locate and contact other family members or caring people outside the family who have the senior's best interest in mind.

The second rule, which amended Rule 4512, requires brokerage firms to make reasonable efforts to obtain the name and contact information of a trusted contact person. A trusted contact person is someone the brokerage firm is authorized to contact and to whom the firm can disclose information about the customer's account to address possible financial exploitation. This is not to be someone who is authorized to make investment or trading decisions for the customer. As FINRA noted in its 2015 rule proposal:

> FINRA intends the trusted contact person to be a resource for the firm in administering the customer's account and in responding to possible financial exploitation. The proposed rule would require that the trusted contact person be age 18 or older and not be authorized to transact business on behalf of the account. A firm may elect to notify an individual that he or she was named as a trusted contact person; however, the proposed rule would not require notification [24].

A trusted contact can be another person the firm can reach out to as an additional layer of protection for a senior investor.

What Is SIFMA Doing?

SIFMA is working collaboratively with policymakers, academic experts, psychologists, and other key stakeholders to better understand the risks to senior investors and the role that firms and advisers can play regarding protecting their investments. While there are many rules which limit an investment professional's ability to take certain actions, SIFMA is working with the investment professionals in attempting to address these limitations and craft new solutions for addressing financial exploitation of older persons.

As these new rules are implemented (such as FINRA Rule 2165 and 4512), work also advances in putting together regional workshops to help firms coordinate with prosecutors, adult protective services, and other firms within their region to jointly and comprehensively address overlapping issues and concerns in this area. The best solution to addressing this problem is to bring together all the people who interact with older investors to create a supportive and protective environment.

SIFMA has also created the Senior Investor Protection Toolkit which is a collection of resources that SIFMA developed several years ago. This document is regularly updated and available for free on the SIFMA website [25] and includes a book identifying the most popular known scams, a one-pager on identifying signs of cognitive decline, and FAQs (frequently asked questions) and other information important to individuals working with seniors. Several other organizations also partnered to develop multiple areas of the toolkit, including AARP (American Association of Retired Persons) and WISER (Women Investing for a Secure Retirement).

One key factor in limiting future exploitation is overcoming the fear that older persons have of a decline in their ability to detect and avoid financial exploitation.

One poll revealed that two thirds of people over 50 are scared of developing dementia, while just 10% are scared of cancer [26]. This may cause elders to "shut down" in order to avoid thinking that they may be at risk for or experiencing dementia-related memory problems, a thought that may cause them pain. In addition, the "overconfidence bias" that may be present in this population may also lead to an overestimate of an older person's own abilities (despite the presence of subjective or objective information suggesting the presence of cognitive impairment), including their ability to avoid financial exploitation [27].

One way to overcome fear and the overconfidence bias is to present information to at-risk persons and empower them to recognize and report exploitation of family and friends. When SIFMA created its toolkit, its emphasis was on educating older individuals about potential scams that could be avoided. Among the things SIFMA has learned through working with other advocacy organizations is that this population is willing to learn about scams if they are doing so to help others (rather than for themselves). Discussing this topic in the context of how others can be helped (instead of yourself) can be useful in avoiding the trigger of resistance and fear.

SIFMA participates in the National Institute of Elder Financial Exploitation (NIEFE) which was created by NAPSA (the National Adult Protective Services Association) to bring together all the many different stakeholders working to address these problems. NIEFE helps pull together an annual event as part of World Elder Abuse Awareness Day, as well as a Financial Exploitation Summit as part of the annual NAPSA Conference, in order to address the issues related to financial exploitation. SIFMA sponsors these activities as well and helps bring various speakers to these programs.

What Doctors Can Do: Case Revisited

Let's go back to our story about Deborah. Suppose she had been suffering from mild cognitive impairment. If someone at the assisted living facility or at her financial institution had been aware of that fact, then they would have been proactively looking for scams against Deborah. In this case, money was kept from going out the door. But there are many examples where these situations are only discovered after the assets have left the institution.

Medical professionals, who have insight into a person's health and cognitive status, have the opportunity to discuss this issue with their patients, include discussions about their financial status when making decisions about healthcare and future planning regarding residence, and surrogate decision-makers. Given the potential impact that these memory issues, even mild cognitive impairment, may have on their decision-making and potentially their financial status, screening and identification of memory problems should be considered. These medical professionals should also encourage their older patients to bring in a trusted contact to help them work through these issues.

References

1. Garcia A. This is the median net worth by age – how do you compare? 2019. Available at https://www.bankrate.com/personal-finance/median-net-worth-by-age/.
2. SIFMA Senior Investor Protection Initiative Client Protection Playbook. Available at https://www.sifma.org/wp-content/uploads/2017/07/toolkit-client-protection-playbook.pdf. https://www.sifma.org/resources/general/senior-investor-protection-toolkit/.
3. CFPB. Reporting of Suspected Elder Financial Exploitation by Financial Institutions. 2019. Available at https://files.consumerfinance.gov/f/documents/cfpb_suspected-elder-financial-exploitation-financial-institutions_report.pdf.
4. The Red Flags of Financial Exploitation and Cognitive Decline, available at https://www.sifma.org/wp-content/uploads/2017/07/toolkit-red-flags-aarp-no-logo.pdf.
5. FDIC Examination Manual Explanation of GLBA Privacy Provisions at: https://www.fdic.gov/regulations/compliance/manual/8/viii-1.1.pdf.
6. 15 U.S.C. § 6802.
7. Fed. Reserve, CFTC, CFPB, FDIC, FTC, NCUA, OCC & SEC. Interagency Guidance on Privacy Laws and Reporting Financial Abuse of Older Adults. 2013. Available at https://files.consumerfinance.gov/f/201309_cfpb_elder-abuse-guidance.pdf.
8. Fed. Reserve, CFTC, CFPB, FDIC, FTC, NCUA, OCC & SEC. Interagency Guidance on Privacy Laws and Reporting Financial Abuse of Older Adults. 2013. Available at https://files.consumerfinance.gov/f/201309_cfpb_elder-abuse-guidance.pdf.
9. https://www.napsa-now.org/wp-content/uploads/2019/10/Guidelines-Bank-Protocol-and-Form-FINAL.1-September-2019-1.pdf.
10. CFPB. Reporting of Suspected Elder Financial Exploitation by Financial Institutions, at 6.
11. Washington State SSB 5042 at https://www.dshs.wa.gov/node/29143.
12. https://www.nasaa.org/industry-resources/senior-issues/model-act-to-protect-vulnerable-adults-from-financial-exploitation/. Laws adopted in other states vary significantly. *See, e.g.,* Florida statute, Fla. Stat. § 825.103, available at http://www.leg.state.fl.us/Statutes/index.cfm?App_mode=Display_Statute&URL=0800-0899/0825/Sections/0825.103.html; Illinois Elder Abuse and Neglect Act, 320 ILCS 20 et seq.
13. https://www.fincen.gov/resources/advisories/fincen-advisory-fin-2011-a003.
14. https://www.justice.gov/elderjustice/eappa-data-overview.
15. https://www.consumerfinance.gov/practitioner-resources/resources-for-older-adults/.
16. https://www.consumer.ftc.gov/blog/2019/10/scams-and-older-consumers-looking-data.
17. https://www.justice.gov/usao/page/file/1121446/download.
18. https://www.justice.gov/elderjustice.
19. 2018. Available at https://www.sec.gov/files/elder-financial-exploitation.pdf
20. 2019. Available at https://www.sec.gov/files/how-the-sec-works-to-protect-senior-investors.pdf.
21. https://www.sec.gov/files/IB%20Help%20for%20APS%20Seniors%20508.pdf.
22. National Senior Investor Initiative, A Coordinated Series of Examinations. Available at https://www.sec.gov/ocie/reportspubs/sec-finra-national-senior-investor-initiative-report.pdf.
23. SEC 2019 Examination Priorities, Office of Compliance Inspections and Examinations, available at https://www.sec.gov/files/OCIE%202019%20Priorities.pdf; FINRA 2019 Annual Risk Monitoring and Examination Priorities Letter, available at https://www.finra.org/rules-guidance/communications-firms/2019-annual-risk-monitoring-and-examination-priorities-letter.
24. FINRA Regulatory Notice 15-37. Available at https://www.finra.org/rules-guidance/notices/15-37.
25. www.sifma.org/seniorinvestortoolkit.
26. https://www.telegraph.co.uk/news/health/elder/11008905/Older-people-are-more-scared-of-dementia-than-cancer-poll-finds.html.
27. Daniel Kahneman, Thinking Fast and Slow, 261-265 (Farrar Straus and Giroux 2011); https://www.behavioraleconomics.com/resources/mini-encyclopedia-of-be/overconfidence-effect/.

Chapter 10
Documentation Practices

Georgia J. Anetzberger and Carol A. Miller

The Role of Healthcare Professionals in Addressing Financial Exploitation

Elder abuse is seen as a major problem for older Americans, widespread and complex, assuming various forms, occurring across settings, and involving many possible perpetrators. However, nowhere are these characteristics more pronounced than with "financial exploitation" (the illegal or improper use of an older adult's money or property), the elder abuse form which has captured media attention and become the "hot issue" for public and private sector activity in recent years. In 2017 the Centers for Disease Control and Prevention recognized financial exploitation of older adults as a serious public health problem. It should not be surprising. Research suggests that financial exploitation may be the most commonly experienced form, whether older adults live in the community or residential care settings [1–4]. Prevalence findings from a review of studies found that healthcare professionals who work with older adults are likely to encounter patients who are victims of elder financial abuse "on a routine basis," since approximately 1 of every 18 cognitively intact older adults living in community settings was affected by financial fraud and scams each year [3]. Its potential perpetrators are far-ranging and may include strangers, businesses, or formal service providers but more often are family members, friends, or neighbors [1].

Beyond these characteristics of financial exploitation are its consequences for victims and society, from lost assets and emotional distress for individuals to increased

G. J. Anetzberger (✉)
Schools of Applied Social Sciences and Medicine, Case Western Reserve University, Cleveland, OH, USA
e-mail: gja3@case.edu

C. A. Miller
Care and Counseling, Brecksville, OH, USA

R. M. Factora (ed.), *Aging and Money*,
https://doi.org/10.1007/978-3-030-67565-3_10

costs of health, justice, and other programs for governments [5, 6]. As a healthcare issue, elder financial exploitation is associated with increased mortality, hospitalizations, functional impairment, and poor physical and mental health [6, 7]. Healthcare professionals, especially those on the frontline in providing services to older adults, can and should assume leadership roles in elder abuse identification, documentation, prevention, treatment, and referral for intervention. This is important for several reasons. First, healthcare professionals are likely to be identified as mandatory reporters in Adult Protective Services (APS) or elder abuse reporting laws nationwide (all states but one have mandatory reporting laws, and all states include financial exploitation as either a stand-alone form or included within another form that must be reported). Second, healthcare professionals are uniquely able to observe changes in the physical, cognitive, or emotional health of their patients and identify signs or indicators of elder abuse in either clinical settings or the victim's home, as in the case of visiting physicians, nurses, therapists, and medical social workers. Third, older adults can be isolated, and healthcare professionals in home or clinical settings may be a primary outside contact. They also tend to trust such professionals and may be willing to share information, usually kept confidential, such as concerns about financial exploitation [8]. Fourth, healthcare professionals can offer needed assistance and guidance to patients/victims or their caregivers. Last, and perhaps most importantly, healthcare professionals have opportunities to identify and document evidence of financial exploitation and other abuse forms and initiate interventions, including referrals, to prevent or halt the abuse. In situations of elder abuse, including financial exploitation, this translates into clinical management of the problem across five phases or steps: detection, assessment, planning, intervention, and follow-up. Documentation is critical throughout these five phases, as discussed in this chapter.

Importance of Documentation by Healthcare Professionals

Documentation represents the recording of observed or reported instances of elder abuse as well as the "suspicion" of probable signs of its occurrence. Documentation can counter denial or support suspicions, which is common in situations of elder abuse and can come from varied sources, even victims and other professionals. It is also essential for communicating with various professionals who are involved with the patient's care as may occur in multidisciplinary teams, widely considered a hallmark for effective elder abuse assessment and intervention [9].With the increasing use of technology-based interprofessional communication (e.g., through e-mail and electronic medical records), it is imperative that each healthcare professional document observations that may be indicative of financial exploitation.

Of the various elder abuse forms, documentation is especially important for financial exploitation, primarily because the investigation could lead to legal proceedings. Observations or standard evaluations contained in the patient's clinical record can serve as evidence if the financial exploitation is prosecuted or surrogate decision-making, like guardianship, is sought for an older adult whose cognitive or mental incapacity renders him/her unable to handle personal finances. Even in situations that

Table 10.1 Examples of professional expertise pertinent to financial exploitation

Observation	Healthcare professional
Mental status decline	Medical, nursing, and mental health professionals
Functional decline	Occupational and physical therapists
Family relationship issues	Social service workers
Lack of necessary medicines or medical equipment	Medical and nursing professionals
Inadequate dietary intake	Registered dieticians

do not involve legal actions, the observations in clinical records can support the voluntary resolution of the financial exploitation. In court situations, if the clinical record and testimony are in conflict, the former may be regarded as more credible. In these contexts, attorneys challenging documentation are likely to consider such recording improprieties or inadequacies as alterations, unprofessional remarks, contradictions, omissions, and opinions, underscoring the importance of healthcare professionals adhering to quality documentation standards (see related section below).

Documentation also is a way of providing observations from objective professionals who base them on their clinical expertise. Although there is a significant overlap in the responsibility of professionals to observe and document clinical indicators of financial exploitation, each healthcare professional has expertise in certain aspects, as summarized in Table 10.1.

Last, documentation can be critical in avoiding liability situations. For example, family members may accuse a healthcare professional of failing to report suspected financial exploitation, in violation of state mandatory elder abuse reporting laws. Actions taken and documented in the clinical record can show that reporting did occur, when, by, and to whom. In addition, since healthcare professionals are legally and ethically required to follow established standards of practice and codes of ethics, documentation supports their having met these obligations. Financial exploitation situations can be particularly complex and ethically challenging, with dilemmas common across such principles as autonomy and beneficence, justice, and nonmaleficence.

Key Qualities of Effective Documentation

To produce the greatest benefit for reporting, preventing, and treating elder abuse, including financial exploitation, documentation must possess eight qualities. Missing even one quality diminishes credibility and limits the usefulness of information being recorded:

1. *Timely:* Documentation should be contemporaneous, undertaken during or immediately after clinical contact, when recall is maximal.
2. *Factual:* Observations must be recorded precisely and objectively, with detail and without interpretation. Care must be taken to avoid words that could com-

promise an investigation or prosecution, such as "alleged financial exploitation" instead of "the patient stated that her home care aide took cash from her purse last week." To the extent possible, documentation should use the patient's own words, placed in quotation marks.

3. *Consistent:* Sections of the clinical record should be consistent.
4. *Organized:* Information should be presented logically and systematically.
5. *Professional:* Documentation must follow discipline-specific standards or formats.
6. *Complete:* Documentation must be thorough, without gaps or omissions.
7. *Routine:* Documentation must be undertaken in the context of "business as usual." Standardized forms and evidence-based instruments should be used where appropriate, such as tools employed during detection and assessment.
8. *Properly stored:* Documentation must be appropriately stored and access limited to professional staff. Its format should ensure that the documentation is durable and readily retrievable.

Content of Documentation

When considering clinical content to document that might be pertinent, it is helpful to think in terms of the following types of conditions associated with risk factors for financial exploitation [10, 11]:

- Vulnerability or dependency by virtue of physical, emotional, cognitive, or other limitations
- Trusting relationship with someone who portrays characteristics of a perpetrator, such as substance abuse or history of violence
- Social isolation
- Controlling relationship or lack of concern by a person on whom the older adult depends
- Questionable ethical foundation of financial transactions
- Secretiveness
- Questionable change of assets

Documentation of financial exploitation and any other accompanying elder abuse forms ideally includes all of the information listed below. It should be noted that some information may seem less relevant to financial exploitation, like environmental data or findings from the physical examination. However, such information can suggest the effects of the loss of income or assets due to financial exploitation along with other accompanying mistreatment:

- Date, time, and setting of patient contact
- Patient demographics, including age, marital status, contact information, and insurance

- Patient's chief complaint and description of any mistreatment
- Behavioral observations, such as cognitive and mental status, interaction between the caregiver and perpetrator (if present), and indications of fear, withdrawal, or agitation
- Caregiver data, including age, gender, cognitive and mental status, financial status, and history of psychotic illness, substance abuse, criminal activity, or violence
- Clinical history, such as chronic medical conditions, medications, functional status, alcohol or drug abuse, and prior hospital admissions
- Relevant social history, like financial situation and its management, living arrangements, and social support
- Environment data (in the case of home visits), including hoarding, vermin, broken locks or windows, and lack of utilities
- Findings from the physical examination, such as patient hygiene, nutrition, and injuries
- Laboratory and diagnostic procedure results, such as a toxicology screen to detect substance abuse, blood urea nitrogen to detect hydration, or X-rays to detect fractures
- Photo documentation and body diagrams of injuries, with notation of such key data as type, number, location, size, and shape as well as explanation given and possible causes
- Opinion on whether the elder abuse was adequately explained
- Interventions carried out and patient's responses
- Follow-up and referral plans, including fulfilling elder abuse reporting requirements

Documentation Across the Five Phases of Clinical Management

Detection

Detection means that a healthcare professional makes a decision about whether or not financial exploitation (or another elder abuse form) is known or suspected in a situation involving an older adult, current patient, or one referred for assessment. The problem is known if examples of it are observed or reported by the older adult or a reliable third party, such as the patient stating that her daughter forged her signature on checks. The problem is suspected if there are possible signs or indicators of its occurrence, such as inability to pay for treatment on the part of the patient when historically this was not the case. In the many situations in which healthcare professionals do not have ongoing contacts with an older adult, it is important to document clues that point toward possible financial exploitation, because these clues may accumulate to build a case for reporting. For example, a hospital-based physical therapist may perform an assessment in preparation for discharge to a skilled care facility, and the patient may make a statement such as: "I have wanted to hire someone to come in and help me with my meals and laundry, but my son handles all my money and he says I cannot afford to have any help. My husband left me with some good resources, so I don't know why I can't afford the help I want." While such a statement may not require a report to APS, it should be documented along with a note about suggesting further evaluation. Such documentation by several professionals across settings and over time may provide evidence to justify reporting for APS investigation.

Screening tools aid in the detection process, formalizing inquiry and ensuring that examples and signs are not overlooked. For example, if a healthcare professional suspects that a patient is being financially exploited, using a simple tool to detect this may be useful (see section on suggested tools). When healthcare professionals do not have access to tools or the expertise to use them, they can initiate a referral for further evaluation. For instance, when medical or nursing professionals note that a patient has difficulty processing information or expresses confusion about money management, they can refer the patient for a geriatric assessment of financial capacity.

Assessment

Assessment goes beyond a simple detection of the abuse. It involves using tools to conduct a thorough evaluation of the problem as well as peripheral issues that could be related to it. For instance, a healthcare professional could assess an older patient's deterioration in cognitive functioning using the Mini-Mental State Examination or the Montreal Cognitive Assessment and its ramifications for independent living and managing finances. Thus, if an initial assessment raises some "red flags" of cognitive decline, it is likely to warrant other layers of assessment using appropriate additional tools (see section on suggested tools). To build on our example of an initial cognitive status assessment, the healthcare professional may need to further investigate the patient's "financial capacity" (functional abilities necessary for handling financial transactions), "consent capacity" (functional abilities needed for decision-making), and "independent living capacity" (skills that enable the individual to live independently and be safe).

The assessment of elder abuse victims and their perpetrators should not be on an ad hoc basis as in our example of assessing the cognitive capacity to live independently and make appropriate financial decisions. Instead it minimally should cover physical health problems, mental and cognitive status changes, functional limitations, financial and environmental issues, recent family or life crises, and diminished social resources [12]. Not only should the healthcare professional list the types of problems identified; he/she should document the frequency with which they occur, their severity, the intent of the perpetrator, and the length of time the abuse has been taking place. In the case of financial exploitation, the healthcare professional could examine the extent to which the victim has been exploited and for how long, its consequences, whether other types of abuse coexist and whether or not the problem has been reported to authorities. Some experts recommend that the assessment focuses on a typical day, the care that the victim needs and receives, and the types of expectations he/she has [13]. All of the information from the assessment process must be documented in the clinical record.

An important point to remember is that the in-depth nature of the assessment will be driven by the type and role of the healthcare professional conducting the assessment. For example, a physician is likely to have less time to conduct a thorough evaluation compared to a social worker or case manager. Sometimes a physician may suspect that financial exploitation is taking place and refer the case to a social worker at the hospital or clinic, who will conduct a more thorough assessment and after that may determine it appropriate to report the case to APS or another authority for investigation.

Furthermore, it may be that the healthcare professional encounters barriers to obtaining necessary information to prepare an appropriate intervention. For instance, healthcare professionals may encounter confidentiality/privacy laws or hesitation from caregivers to divulge needed information on financial exploitation. They also are likely to face barriers in probing about the financial assets of their patients or obtaining protected information from financial advisors or banking officials. Often financial advisors on their part may recognize signs of diminished capacity exhibited by their clients but lack sufficient knowledge to assess that capacity or to develop a course of action to contact healthcare professionals in order to conduct a follow-up. In this sense the lack of trust, privacy issues, or lack of familiarity with each other's role may inhibit effective interactions between healthcare and banking or financial management professionals.

Planning

During planning, documentation details the course of action to be undertaken based upon the assessment. Particularly in instances of financial exploitation, various civil or criminal legal remedies may be considered. However, planning to address elder abuse most likely will involve the selection of appropriate community resources [14, 15]. These may include emergency services, such as crisis hotlines and shelters; support services, like home-delivered meals and adult day care; and rehabilitative services, such as mental health counseling and substance abuse treatment. Locating community resources can be facilitated by using linkage services, like those offering information and referral, including the Eldercare Locator program nationally and Aging and Disability Resource Centers locally.

Intervention

Documentation during the intervention phase involves recording the results of clinical procedures, legal remedies, and interventions employed to address the elder abuse situation or prevent its reoccurrence. In clinical settings, the primary intervention taken by healthcare professionals may be the referral of the case to APS or to a comprehensive geriatric assessment program for further action. It should be mentioned that there is limited evaluative research on interventions to address elder abuse, including financial exploitation, although commitment to rectify this deficiency has increased in recent years. Systematic reviews of published research suggest that to date few studies used high-quality evaluative methods and even fewer interventions demonstrated effectiveness in problem prevention or resolution [16, 17].

Follow-Up

Finally, during this last phase of clinical management, the healthcare professional follows up with the patient/victim and his/her caregiver to evaluate the extent to which the proposed intervention was followed, its effectiveness in helping to resolve and/or prevent a reoccurrence of the problem, and whether a reassessment is necessary. For example, in the case of a victim of financial exploitation who was suffering from depression, it will be important for the healthcare professional to address whether or not the depression is improving.

Examples of Tools to Detect and Assess Financial Exploitation

One simple tool for detecting financial exploitation is a four-item measure that was developed by Quinn and Tomita (1997) [13] and later adapted by Beach et al. (2010) [18]. The four items are as follows: (a) Have you signed anything that you didn't quite understand? (b) Has anyone asked you to sign anything without explaining what you were signing? (c) Has anyone taken your checks without permission? (d) Have you suspected that anyone was tampering with your savings or other assets? The items are coded dichotomously and ask whether it has occurred since turning 60 and specifically in the past 6 months. Those responding "yes" to any of the four questions are considered to have experienced financial exploitation.

Another relevant tool is the Older Adult Financial Exploitation Measure (OAFEM) [19]. The authors tested a 79-item measure as well as shorter versions with 54 and 30 items, all of which had high reliability and validity. Results suggested a single hierarchy of four major constructs in the order of the severity of financial exploitation: major theft and scams, lesser theft and scams, risk, and entitlement and expectations. The short forms excluded items on risk of abuse, since they did not relate to actual financial exploitation. Items from the 30-item measure include the following: (a) Has X become the payee on your benefit check and used the money for themselves (major theft and scams)? (b) Has X persuaded you to sign any documents even though it was not in your best interest (lesser theft and scams)?

Beyond tools that detect or assess financial exploitation are those that evaluate financial decision-making ability. These can be helpful in identifying older adults at potential risk of financial exploitation in order to prevent occurrence of the problem. A set of such tools was developed by Lichtenberg and his colleagues [20]. The Lichtenberg Screening Scale seeks to examine four major aspects of informed financial decision-making and communication: choice, understanding, appreciation, and rationale. It is a rating scale that requires the user to assess the accuracy of an older adult's answers to ten questions, also recording comments made for each question. Sample questions include the following: (a)What is the financial decision you are making/have made? (b) How will the decision impact you now and over time? (c) Who benefits most from the decision?

When a situation indicates the need for a formal evaluation of financial decision-making capacity, healthcare professionals can initiate a referral to a geriatric mental health professional, who would use an evidence-based tool such as the 77-question Lichtenberg Financial Decision-Making Rating Scale [21]. The Scale has been adapted as a 13-item Family and Friends Scale [22] that can serve as a guide for healthcare professionals to document concerns about a patient's financial capacity as in the following sample questions: (a) Does the patient seem anxious or distressed regarding their financial decisions and/or transactions? (b) Does the patient rely on one person for financial decisions?

The routine completion of tools to detect financial exploitation or assess financial decision-making ability and their inclusion in the clinical record improves and standardizes documentation. When healthcare professionals do not have access to evidence-based tools, or when it is not within the scope of their practice to use a formal tool, they can document their recommendation that the patient be evaluated by a professional who is qualified to assess financial capacity.

Challenges in Clinical Settings

With the almost universal use of electronic health records, it is increasingly difficult to document observations that do not fall within the context of standard forms imbedded in the charting system. Despite this limitation, every healthcare professional has the ability – and the responsibility – to document a narrative note describ ing any observation of or statement made by an older adult in a clinical setting that may be an indicator of or clue to financial exploitation. Many older adults who receive care in large healthcare systems are seen by numerous professionals with little in-person continuity among the healthcare providers and much of the "coordination" occurring by someone who does "case management" either by phone or by reviewing the documentation. Thus, it is imperative that each healthcare professional documents information from his/her professional perspective so the "pieces of the puzzle" can be put together in situations of elder financial exploitation. The following case example illustrates how a visiting nurse was able to document those pieces during several visits and advocate for actions to protect an older adult.

Case Example: Visiting Nurse Documents Financial Exploitation

First Skilled Nursing Visit

Gertrude still lives in the home in which she was born 86 years ago, in a rural county in the Midwest. Gertrude has been hospitalized several times during the last year for unstable heart failure, and she now receives skilled nursing care. During Nurse Samantha's first visit, Gertrude said she was ashamed of the rundown condition of her house, stating she had been in and out of the hospital so much she could never follow through with plans for repairs. Nurse Samantha noted that buckets were placed in several rooms to catch the water from leaks in the ceilings. Windows were old and did not close tightly, and the water was turned off to the bathtub.

Gertrude told Nurse Samantha that "a nice young man—I think his name was Bill—stopped by about a month ago and said he was certified by the county office on aging to do home repair work. He told me he was a good friend of Susan, the person who delivers my meals on wheels. He said that the office on aging has a special fund to pay for home repairs for senior citizens who have lived in their homes for at least 25 years and that I would only have to pay $5,000 for new windows and roofing materials. Well, he cashed my check and then I ended up in the hospital and he hasn't come around again. He didn't leave a phone number, but he told me I could get in touch with him through Susan, so I'll ask her about him the next time I see her."

Nursing documentation THe patient's house in rundown condition with water dripping through ceilings, no running water in bathtub, and windows in disrepair. The patient reported that she wrote a check for $5000 about a month ago and gave it to a man (Bill?) who promised to do repairs. Upon further questioning, the patient said she will ask Susan, who works for the county meals on wheels program, about contact information so she can get the work done as promised.

Subsequent Skilled Nursing Visits

During each of the next few visits, Nurse Samantha asked Gertrude about any success with getting contact information for Bill. Each time Gertrude said she kept forgetting to ask Susan, but she was confident that Bill would be bringing the windows as soon as the weather got warmer. Nurse Samantha planned her fourth visit to coincide with Susan's visit, and she reminded Gertrude to ask about Bill. Susan declared, "I never heard of Bill until a couple of the people on my delivery route told me about him asking them for money for home repairs. I asked Paul, our center director, about this and he told me that a man named Bill used to work in the maintenance department but was fired for stealing supplies from our department."

Nursing documentation and actions Met Susan, from the county office on aging, at the patient's house and found out that the man who cashed the patient's $5000 check for home repairs a couple months ago and did not return may be a former employee, named Bill, who was fired for stealing. Incident was reported to nursing supervisor, and a report was filed with county APS agency. Physician was contacted to request order for medical social service worker to visit patient and evaluate the need for comprehensive geriatric assessment.

References

1. Acierno R, Hernandez MA, Amstader AB, et al. Prevalence and correlates of emotional, physical, sexual, neglectful, and financial abuse in the United States. Am J Public Health. 2010;100:292–7.
2. Peterson JC, Burnes DPR, Caccamise PL, et al. Financial exploitation of older adults: a population-prevalence study. J Gen Intern Med. 2014;29:1615–23.
3. Burnes D, Henderson CR Jr, Sheppard C, Zhao R, Pillemer K, Lachs MS. Prevalence of financial fraud and scams among older adults in the United States: a systematic review and meta-analysis. Am J Public Health. 2017;107(8):e13–21.
4. Page C, Conner T, Prokharov A, Fang Y, Post L. The effect of care setting on elder abuse: results from a Michigan survey. J Elder Abuse Negl. 2009;21:239–52.
5. MetLife Mature Market Institute, National Committee for the Prevention of Elder Abuse, Virginia Tech, University of Kentucky. The MetLife study of elder financial abuse: crimes of occasion, desperation, and predation against America's elders. New York: Metropolitan Life Insurance Company; 2011.
6. Weissberger GH, Mosqueda L, Nguyen A, et al. Physical and mental health correlates of perceived financial exploitation in older adults: preliminary findings from the Finance, Cognitive, and Health in Elders Study (FINCHES). Aging Ment Health. 2009; https://doi.org/10.1080/13607863.2019.1571020.
7. Acierno R, Watkins J, Hernandez-Tejada MA, et al. Mental health correlates of financial mistreatment in the National Elder Mistreatment Study Wave II. J Aging Health. 2018;31(7):1196–211.
8. Miller CA. Elder abuse and nursing: what nurses need to know and can do about it. New York: Springer; 2017.
9. Anetzberger GJ. Elder abuse multidisciplinary teams. In: Dong Y, editor. Elder abuse: research, practice and policy. Cham: Switzerland. Springer Nature; 2017. p. 417–32.
10. Pham E, Liao S. Clinicians role in the documentation of elder mistreatment. Geriatr Aging. 2009;12(6):323–7.
11. Kemp BJ, Mosqueda LA. Elder financial abuse: an evaluation framework and supporting evidence. J Am Geriatr Soc. 2005;53:1123–7.
12. Anetzberger GJ. Clinical management of elder abuse: general considerations. Clin Gerontol. 2005;28(1/2):27–41.

13. Quinn MJ, Tomito SK. Elder abuse and neglect: causes, diagnosis, and intervention strategies. 2nd ed. New York: Springer; 1997.
14. Jackson SL. Understanding elder abuse: a clinician's guide. Washington, DC: American Psychological Association; 2018.
15. Anetzberger GJ. Intersection of public health and nontraditional partners and approaches to address elder abuse. In: Teaster PB, Hall JE, editors. Elder abuse and the public's health. New York: Springer; 2018. p. 125–51.
16. Rosen T, Elman A, Dion S, et al. Review of programs to combat elder mistreatment: focus on hospitals and level of resources needed. J Am Geriatr Soc. 2019;67(6):1286–94.
17. Ploeg J, Hutchison B, MacMillan H, Bolan G. A systematic review of interventions for elder abuse. J Elder Abuse Negl. 2009;21:187–210.
18. Beach SR, Schulz R, Castle NG, Rosen J. Financial exploitation and psychological mistreatment among older adults: differences between African Americans and non-African Americans in population-based survey. Gerontologist. 2010;50(6):744–57.
19. Conrad KJ, Iris M, Ridings W, Langley K, Wilber KH. Self-report measure of financial exploitation of older adults. Gerontologist. 2010;50(6):758–73.
20. Lichtenberg PA, Howard H, Simaskp P, et al. The Lichtenberg financial decision screening scale (LFDSS): a new tool for assessing financial decision-making and preventing financial exploitation. J Elder Abuse Negl. 2016;28(3):134–51.
21. Lichtenberg PA, Stoltman J, Ficker LJ, Iris M, Mast B. A person-centered approach to financial capacity assessment: preliminary development of a new rating scale. Clin Gerontol. 2015;38(1):49–67.
22. Campbell RC, Lichtenberg PA, Hall LN, Teresi JA, Ocepek-Welikson K. Assessment of financial decision-making: an informant scale. J Elder Abuse Negl. 2019;31(2):115–28.

Chapter 11
Addressing Senior Financial Abuse: Adult Protective Services and Other Community Resources

Jason Burnett, Sharlene Nauls, Lori Albee, and Renee J. Flores

Chapter Overview

Annually, millions of seniors are targeted and fall victim to financial abuse (i.e., financial exploitation, frauds, and scams) [1]. The consequences are wide-ranging and often detrimental both financially and personally [2–4]. Across the United States (US), these heinous acts are being met with focused federal, state, and community assistance and resources to prevent their occurrence, mitigate the impacts, and promote recovery and resilience for those affected [5] [6]. Creating awareness of these available resources is critical for stemming the tide of senior financial abuse in the United States. This chapter highlights agencies and organizations working to create communities where seniors are protected from financial crimes and their impact. The primary focus is on the role that frontline agencies such as Adult Protective Services (APS) and their community partners play to assist with keeping seniors safe.

J. Burnett (✉) · R. J. Flores
Internal Medicine, Division of Geriatric and Palliative Medicine, The University of Texas Health Science Center at Houston, (UTHealth), McGovern Medical School, Houston, TX, USA
e-mail: Jason.Burnett@uth.tmc.edu; Renee.J.Flores@uth.tmc.edu

S. Nauls · L. Albee
The Texas Department of Family and Protective Services, Adult Protective Services, Houston, TX, USA
e-mail: Sharlene.Nauls@dfps.state.tx.us; Lori.Albee2@dfps.state.tx.us

R. M. Factora (ed.), *Aging and Money*,
https://doi.org/10.1007/978-3-030-67565-3_11

Financial Abuse at a Glance

Scenario 1

Imagine that your parents are retired and dependent on their social security and a savings account worth $200,000.00 to support them for the remainder of their lives. Although minimal, they need assistance with grocery shopping, cooking, cleaning, and paying the bills. You live out of state. They want to remain living in their own home so they hire a daily caregiver. The relationship seems to be built on mutual trust and benefit. Your parents give the caregiver access to the bank account and other financial resources to purchase food and pay the bills. Since the caregiver arrived, you don't hear from your parents as often, even if you call. When you do talk to them, they say everything is fine. After a few months, you visit and find their home is extremely unkempt, and they are living with minimal food. Upon further inspection you find that their savings account has been depleted and the caregiver has quit.

Scenario 2

Your grandfather lives alone. When visiting, you see a bank statement showing several bank transfers of $5000.00 over the past couple of months totaling $20,000.00. As a result he is falling behind on his bills and facing eviction from his apartment. When you ask, he does not remember what he did with the money, but while visiting her receives a call from a recent "acquaintance" he made over the Internet. You request that he allows you to manage his finances and he vehemently refuses. Sometime later, you receive a phone call from his apartment complex stating that he is being evicted due to nonpayment.

These two scenarios, among many others, occur daily in the United States, and those affected (i.e., victims, family members, etc.) are left asking questions such as the following: Who do I call? Is there an agency, service, or resource that could help get restitution for my parents or grandfather? Are there services to help my parents or grandfather manage their money so that they are not exploited again? Are there programs for helping get protections in place such as allowing me or some other trusted family member to take over the financial decisions for my parents or grandfather despite their reluctance? Most importantly, how could these acts have been prevented? Fortunately, there are programs and services spread throughout communities to assist with prevention, detection, and response to senior financial abuse.

Community Resources and Networks

No single entity is sufficient to address senior financial abuse. Robust responses require partnerships between public and private organizations that provide varying resources. Leveraging community resources through networks to address elder abuse issues including financial abuse has increased stakeholder coordination, public awareness, and criminal and legal actions all leading to better prevention, detection, and responses [7].

Nationally, there is an estimated 891 formal elder abuse networks that address senior financial abuse spread out over the 3143 US counties. This represents a coverage area of only 25% of counties. Even fewer counties (2%) have networks which focus all of their resources on senior financial abuse (6%). Most networks, including those focusing exclusively on senior financial abuse, are located in densely populated cities rather than areas with the highest population density of seniors [7]. This limits the availability and accessibility of important resources for many seniors experiencing or at risk for financial abuse; especially those living in rural areas where senior populations are growing the fastest and yet continue to suffer from limited resources and senior support. Fortunately, there are some senior resources such as Adult Protective Services (APS) and law enforcement that cover all 3143 counties.

Adult Protective Services

Purpose

Adult Protective Services (APS) are agencies across the United States that respond to allegations of abuse, neglect, and exploitation of vulnerable adults, including seniors. These programs are conceptually equivalent to child protective services [8]. APS programs were developed as a result of a federal mandate attached to Title XX of the 1975 Social Security Act which formalized a national response to adult abuse. The majority of APS programs are funded by social service block grants and state generated revenue funds [9]. Located in all 50 states as well as the US territories of Guam, Puerto Rico, and the Virgin Islands, APS provides senior support in all 3143 counties making them the most available non-law enforcement agency for addressing financial abuse in seniors.

Financial Abuse Definitions

Through the federal mandate, APS agencies were given latitude to develop their own policies and practices regarding which types of abuse they would investigate and how they would investigate and respond to reportable abuse. To date, every APS program receives and investigates allegations of senior financial abuse. Broadly, financial abuse occurs when someone illegally or dishonestly uses another person's money for their own benefit [10]. Each program has specific state statues that define financial abuse, therefore providing parameters around the types of financial abuse the program accepts for investigation and for service provision. For example, some states only investigate financial abuse occurring when the beneficiary is a person of "trust." This excludes most instances of fraud and scams. Other programs include any type of financial abuse regardless of the relationship between the alleged victim and alleged perpetrator. The best way to determine which definition is used in a state or county is to review the respective online elder abuse statutes.

Allegation Reporting

Anyone can report a suspected case of financial abuse to APS. However, all states have established mandatory reporting laws specifying which community members are required to make reports. In some states such as Texas, all "capable" adults 18 years and older are mandated reporters regardless of pre-existing professional confidentiality guidelines [11]. In other states only professionals working in supportive roles with seniors are required to report suspicion of financial abuse. All APS programs have designated ways for the public to make an anonymous report, and these generally consist of calling an abuse hotline or entering a referral online. The most recently updated reporting laws and methods, in each state at the time of this writing, can be found on the American Bar Association's Commission on Law and Aging website [12].

Intake and Investigations

Generally, investigations begin with intake screening against statutory guidelines. The referred allegations must meet the state-specific definition for the type of abuse as well as meet any guidelines related to age. For example, some states require individuals <64 years of age to have a documented disability in order to be investigated for financial or any other type of abuse. Referrals meeting the guidelines get screened in and receive an investigation within a timeframe linked to the level of urgency for preventing ongoing or future harm. Therefore, someone facing impoverishment or restriction of basic needs such as medical care, food, or shelter as a result of financial abuse will have a shorter investigation initiation timeframe. Nationally, investigations begin (i.e., initial agency contact with the alleged victim) anywhere from ≤24 hours up to 20 days with most programs responding between 2 and 10 days [9].

APS conducts evidence-based driven investigations. Investigations of financial abuse often include face-to-face visits in the senior's home to conduct a needs assessment and collect varying levels of socioecological data related to the case. In financial abuse cases, banking and other financial records are collected from the senior and requested from the relevant financial institution(s). When allowable under federal and state statutes, the ability to request and receive financial records from financial institutions is a strength of APS programs. These data along with interviews and other supplemental case information are critical for determining the validity of the allegation. Seventy-five percent of APS programs require a preponderance of evidence (≥51%) to validate an allegation of financial abuse. This information is also used as supporting evidence in cases that result in criminal investigations and legal remedies.

Resource Linkage and Service Delivery

The networks APS forms with senior community resources are vital to their mission which is to keep seniors safe from further financial abuse and its detriments. APS does this primarily by linking seniors who have been financially abused to community resources and services that can assist with further protection, replenishment of lost funds or property, or other needs that may have arisen due to victimization. Most APS programs form strong partnerships with local and state law enforcement agencies to assist with senior protection. An APS-validated allegation of financial abuse is considered evidence of a crime in most states and therefore results in a referral to local law enforcement for criminal investigation. When dealing with fraud and scams, the case may be referred to the State Attorneys General Office – Consumer Protection Division or Medicaid Fraud Control Units, to federal agencies such as the Federal Bureau of Investigation for web-based fraud/scams, or to the United States Postal Inspection Service when the fraud or scam occurs through the mail. For a short list of major federal agencies responding to senior financial abuse, see Appendix A.

Aside from law enforcement, APS has strong community partnerships and often makes referrals to a variety of senior-serving organizations. In cases where financial abuse has led to food insecurity, a referral may be made to meals on wheels or to the local food bank. To assist with ongoing financial protection, a senior may be linked to daily money management programs or guardianship programs when the senior is believed to be unable to adequately manage his/her finances. These resources and services are aimed at providing immediate and long-term protection from financial abuse and related consequences. To learn more about APS programs across the United States, visit the National Adult Protective Services Association website [13], and to learn the specific flow chart for APS referrals and responses, view the National Center on Elder Abuse APS flow diagram [14].

APS Case 1

The victim was a 75-year-old female. Her caregiver took three checks from her checkbook and wrote them to herself totaling $2500. Within a month, the victim realized the checks were missing and filed a fraud claim with the bank as well as a police report. The police made a referral to APS who was able to obtain evidence from the police report and bank records showing the caregiver had forged the victim's signature and deposited the money into a personal account. This collective evidence was enough for APS to reach the determination that the caregiver, without the consent of the senior, took money and benefited personally. The APS case investigation data was shared with law enforcement, and the caregiver was charged with forgery. The charge was increased to a third-degree felony due to statutory enhancements for crimes against an elderly person. Additionally, APS placed the caregivers name on the Health and Human Services Commission Employee Misconduct Registry, which ensures that unlicensed personnel who commit acts of abuse, neglect, and exploitation against the elderly and people with disabilities are denied employment in regulated facilities and agencies. Restitution was paid to the senior in the amount of $5000.00.

This case, like many others, illustrates the importance of community partnerships for addressing senior financial abuse. Law enforcement during criminal investigations is not likely to request bank records or address social needs of a victim. Therefore, APS was called, and as part of their investigation, they worked with the bank to obtain financial records. This information along with the criminal investigation evidence was then presented to the District Attorney's Office resulting in subsequent prosecution. Without these partnerships, restitution for the senior is much less likely.

APS Case 2

The victim was a 79-year-old male. The perpetrator had power of attorney to manage victim's finances. The perpetrator was using a joint account to pay the victim's bills including the fees for private duty nurse. A family member suspected financial misconduct and reported the case to APS. APS obtained financial records on six personal accounts for the perpetrator and two joint accounts with the victim. The discovery showed millions of dollars in transferred funds from the joint accounts to the perpetrators personal account. Expensive purchases such as cars, jewelry, and property were made by the perpetrator. The victim's medical records showed documented cognitive impairments indicating the inability to provide informed consent prior to the purchases. The finding was that the perpetrator misused his fiduciary power to commit financial abuse. The case was referred to law enforcement and resulted in a criminal investigation, prosecution, and imprisonment. APS worked with the local guardianship program to appoint a guardian and worked with the local probate courts to appoint a new power of attorney to manage the senior's finances.

This case introduces new complexities that require additional community partnerships that include health professionals for medical and decision-making capacity determinations, forensic accountants to track the different accounts over time and spending patterns, as well as guardianship programs to put a guardian in place for the senior to protect him from future abuse.

Law Enforcement

In the cases above, law enforcement served a critical role in protecting the senior by conducting criminal investigations and referring the cases to the county District Attorney's Office for prosecution. This is the main role that law enforcement plays in addressing senior financial abuse. Fortunately, similar to APS, law enforcement agencies serve every US county and are options for reporting suspected financial abuse. The response from these agencies may vary considerably however, depending on the structure of the agency. Agencies located in large metropolitan cities may have a financial crimes division that includes forensic accountants or a special victims division that focuses on crimes involving seniors, but this is less likely to be the case in smaller rural areas. Aforementioned, law enforcement agencies in population-dense cities are more likely to have access to senior networks such as elder abuse multidisciplinary teams and Triads (discussed below) to assist with financial abuse cases. However, a lack of financial crimes expertise within a law enforcement agency should not deter a person from reporting a suspected financial crime against a senior. These agencies often work closely with other local and state law enforcement agencies such as the State Attorneys General Office and may be able to recruit their assistance when needed. Understanding their limitations and the need for a community response, law enforcement agencies across the United States have developed their own networks to increase the safety and well-being of seniors.

Protecting and Serving Seniors of Financial Abuse Through Triads

Triads are community networks that consist specifically of law enforcement, members from the local senior community, and senior community services or resource organizations. Triads place seniors in the center and work to form a safety net around them. Triad goals are generally to reduce crime against seniors and to reduce senior's fear of victimization. They achieve this through Senior and Law Enforcement Together (SALT) councils in which members of the triad generate ideas and actionable initiatives and put those initiatives into action. Including senior perspectives strengthens communications and relationships between seniors and organizations and builds a sense of community where seniors are not forgotten, thereby reducing isolation and other facilitators of financial abuse and expanding law enforcement capabilities within communities. A major communication gap that is bridged by Triads is the cooperation between seniors and law enforcement. Most elder abuse including financial abuse occurs by a family member, creating a situation where the senior may be reluctant to cooperate with a criminal investigation in fear of the family member getting into trouble [15]. Understanding the perspectives of both groups can help reach reasonable alternative solutions that meet the victim's desires and allow law enforcement to do their job.

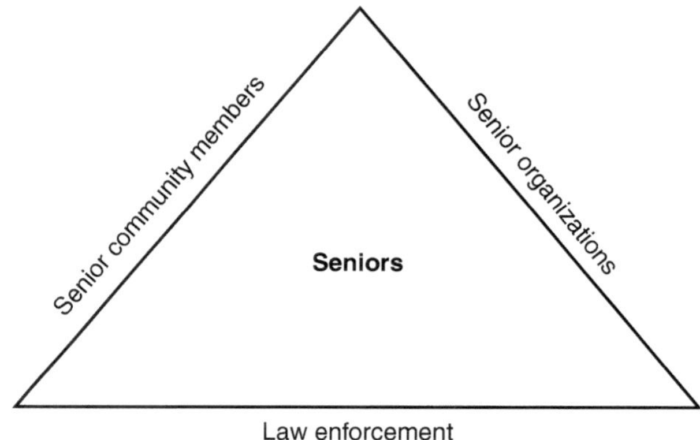

Fig. 11.1 Basic foundation of elder abuse triads

To date, Triads represent over 600 (~70%) of the known elder abuse networks throughout the United States. None are known to work exclusively to address senior financial abuse. For more information on Triads and to locate the nearest one, visit the National Sheriffs' Association of Triads webpage [16] (Fig. 11.1).

Elder Abuse Multidisciplinary Teams

Multidisciplinary teams (MDTs) are significant innovations in the field of elder abuse and are subtly distinct from Triads. MDTs focus more on ensuring robust criminal and legal responses to instances of financial and other forms of abuse. Multiple professionals from organizations such as APS, law enforcement, local and state attorney's offices, medicine, and social work share data and expertise on senior abuse cases with the focus on immediate protection through service linkage and long-term protection through criminal and legal action. The ranking core qualities of an MDT are (1) multiple stakeholders with similar missions (i.e., addressing elder abuse and its consequences); (2) understanding and respect for other stakeholders response pathways, facilitators, barriers, and outcomes; (3) the need for transparent interagency collaborations (i.e., communication) to fully address senior financial abuse; and (4) the willingness to work together to achieve the best case resolution, avoiding blame and shame. Most MDTs simply conduct case reviews to help determine whether a case is valid and to guide the next steps for protecting and serving the senior [17].

Elder Abuse Forensic Centers

Elder abuse forensic centers are MDTs that not only conduct both case reviews but also have the infrastructure to assess the senior. In cases of financial abuse, these centers may conduct standardized cognitive assessments of the senior to determine their ability to manage their finances. They will also conduct forensic interviews to gather additional evidence from the senior, regarding the alleged crime that can be used in legal proceedings. The evidence from elder abuse forensic centers shows increases in protective services through guardianship appointments [18] and improved financial outcomes through prosecutions and victim restitution [19].

Enhanced MDTs

Recent enhancements to elder abuse MDTs have focused specifically on addressing senior financial abuse. These enhanced MDTs (E-MDTs) are now including forensic accounting as a core member to assist with evidence summation and testimony. These enhancements have shown to have great promise for helping seniors get justice and in some cases, more importantly, recovered financial losses. They are particularly helpful in complex financial abuse cases.

Financial Abuse Specialist Teams

Financial abuse specialist teams (FAST) are MDTs that work either within an APS program or within the general community. Those within APS programs provide specialized financial abuse investigative support directly to the APS agency. Members of the team will work the cases along with the APS caseworkers to help detect spending patterns, summate the findings, and present the findings in court if necessary. In the community setting, FAST primarily serves as an educational resource for community organizations regarding scams, fraud, and guidance on here to seek other support for addressing senior financial abuse.

While MDTs are populating across the country as a best practice for financial and elder abuse response, placing these teams in every jurisdiction and making them accessible have not been feasible due to current federal, state, and local community funding and workforce shortages. However, given the shift toward virtual meetings as a result of the COVID-19 pandemic, the availability of these teams to be accessible to more communities throughout the United States may become a new reality. To learn more about elder abuse MDTs and to locate the nearest one, visit the National Institute of Justice Elder Abuse Multidisciplinary Team Resource page [20].

Community-Based Senior Resources

The APS cases above illustrate the need for community partnerships that go beyond an APS and law enforcement collaboration. Financial abuse cases can be complex to investigate, but it can be equally complicated to address the needs of the senior after being victimized. There are a range of needs that may arise including the need for food, legal services, housing, long-term financial decision-making or monitoring, and other needs that may have been diminished. The following community resources provide a range of services that can be sought to meet the varying needs of seniors who fall victim to financial abuse.

Area Agencies on Aging

The 1965 Older Americans Act established aging networks through the development of Area Agencies on Aging [21]. Currently there are approximately 622 Area Agencies on Aging across the United States providing available services in almost every community. The National Association of Area Agencies on Aging (n4a) has teamed up with Wells Fargo Bank to help address senior financial abuse prevention and protection through educational initiatives. In addition AAA provides a range of services that could assist with overcoming the consequences of financial abuse such as locating licensed caregivers and supporting legal issues that may include guardianship, health and long-term care, and public benefit programs. For more information on AAA services, visit the National Association of Area Agencies on Aging website [22] or the Administration for Community Living elder locator webpage [23].

American Association of Retired Persons (AARP)

Financial abuse can have devastating effects on a senior's ability to stay in their homes and pay their bills. AARP is a national organization that provides services to seniors in the form of education and consumer advocacy. This organization can provide legal counsel in financial abuse cases where the victim is facing foreclosure, has experienced real property fraud, faces unrelenting debt collection as a result of financial insecurity, or represents the senior in other general consumer issues that may be affected by financial abuse. As part of their community and professional educational initiatives, the AARP has an established District Collaborative Training and Response for Older Victims focusing on cross-training professionals who encounter older adults to improve detection, investigations, and collaborations on elder abuse cases. For more information on AARP senior services that may assist financial abuse victims, visit the AARP legal counsel and consumer fraud resources page [24].

Better Business Bureaus

Some agencies serve mostly as community education conduits and, therefore, provide indirect financial abuse services. Better Business Bureaus (BBBs) are consumer protection organizations that provide senior protection against financial abuse by cataloguing consumer complaints against businesses and through community education regrading prevalent fraud and scam schemes. They also provide tip sheets and other resources to assist seniors and others with preventing financial abuse. For more information on BBBs, visit the national Better Business Bureau resource page [25].

Daily Money Management Programs

Daily money management (DMM) programs are good ways for seniors to manage their finances, but they may also prevent seniors from being financially abused. DMM programs can help seniors set budgets, automatic drafting, and account passwords and provide other financial support that can assist with financial oversight, routine financial reviews, and account balancing and dispute fraudulent transactions or incorrect bills. These programs have been shown to save seniors' significant amounts of money [26]. For more information on DMM programs or to locate a daily money manager, visit the American Association of Daily Money Management webpage [27].

Faith Organizations

Financial abuse can severely impact seniors psychologically and socially [4, 28]. Faith organizations have been identified as organizations that victims of elder abuse including financial abuse turn to and can provide strong support systems for seniors who may need social and financial support following a crisis [29]. Fortunately, most, if not all, communities have faith organizations that can provide welfare checks on seniors to promote socialization and normalcy following a financial abuse incident. Members of these organizations may also provide monetary, transportation, or meal support for seniors who fall victim to financial abuse and are unable to afford their routine needs.

Financial Institutions

Financial institutions are located in proximity to every community. These institutions often protect the financial security of seniors through fraud protection programs. Financial institutions are required to submit suspicious activity reports to the Consumer Fraud Protection Bureau (see federal agencies in Appendix A for more of the CFPB). In 2018, the Senior Safe Act was passed which gives covered financial institutions' immunity from liability when making reports of suspected senior financial abuse [30]. Often times, banks and other financial institutions will provide financial records to APS, in support of the investigation, when requested. Legislation has also been adopted in several states allowing financial institutions to place time-limited holds on accounts when financial abuse is suspected. More and more financial institutions are also engaging in staff training to detect senior financial abuse as well as community education to raise awareness of the problem.

Guardianship Programs

When a senior is unable to make informed decisions regarding his or her health or finances, it is critical that an advocate is put in place to prevent ongoing or future financial abuse. Senior guardianship programs are designed to provide protection of seniors through court-appointed advocates or guardians. The guardian is expected to make decisions on behalf of the senior and in the best interest of the senior. These decisions often regard healthcare and financial decisions during all stages of life. Guardians are required to provide timely and accurate service reports to the courts. Petitioning for a guardian often occurs through APS after the client is found to lack decision-making capacity or through a legal petition by a family member or court [31].

Legal Services: Prosecutorial, Civil, and Asset Protection

Legal services fall into three categories regarding senior financial abuse. These categories are criminal and civil remedies and asset protection. Most communities have legal representatives that work with local law enforcement to assist with the prosecution, and a family lawyer can likely argue a civil lawsuit in response to financial abuse. Asset protection however may require seeking out specialized legal services such as an elder law attorney. For example, a family member or a senior may wish to prevent financial abuse by establishing a durable power of attorney (POA) or a revocable living trust. Durable POA preemptively establishes a designee to take over management of a person's finances or estate (financial POA) or medical decisions (healthcare POA) if the person becomes incapacitated. A revocable living trust can be set up through an attorney that gives a designee the authority to make financial decisions on behalf of the senior. The senior retains the ability to make decisions, while the revocable living trust is in place as long as they are deemed capable by the courts. They are also allowed to revoke the decision-making of the designee at any time. For more information on legal resources to help prevent and combat senior financial abuse, visit the American Bar Association Commission on Law and Aging website [32].

Meals on Wheels

Financial loss can lead to destitution and poverty severely affecting a senior's ability to afford everyday necessities such as food. The Meals on Wheels of America program supports over 5000 community nutrition programs nationwide that provide seniors with daily healthy meals. This program is needs-based and is paid for through public donations and grants. To learn more or to locate a provider, visit the Meals on Wheels of America website [33].

Although this list of community resources is not exhaustive, it provides some reasonable and available programs to seek services for seniors. Aside from these agencies and organizations, there are also federal agencies and resources for those at risk or affected by financial abuse.

Federal Agencies and Resources

This chapter would be remiss if the federal agencies and resources for addressing senior financial abuse were not mentioned. There has been considerable effort at the federal level to stem the tide of senior financial abuse [5, 6]. Some of the major agencies involved include the Social Security Administration Representative Payee Program, the United States Postal Inspection Service investigations into mail fraud and scams, the Consumer Financial Protection Bureau and Suspicious Activity Reporting, and the Federal Bureau of Investigation's financial and cybercrimes unit. Other federal agencies such as the US Department of Health and Human Services, Administration on Community Living, the US Department of Justice Office for Victims of Crimes, the National Institute of Justice, and the Victims of Crime Act have contributed federal grant funds to assist state and community agencies and organizations to address senior financial abuse. An abbreviated list of major federal agencies and programs with a focus on addressing senior financial abuse is provided in the appendices.

Conclusion

The fast-growing nature of financial abuse has garnered much needed attention and response from federal, state, and local community agencies throughout the United States. Strong networks consisting of APS, law enforcement, seniors, senior organizations, and other professionals have been developed, and evidence from these networks are encouraging for improving protection and outcomes for seniors suffering and/or at risk for financial abuse. Unfortunately, these networks aren't in every community due to funding and workforce shortages. Nevertheless, agencies such as APS and law enforcement who do provide services and resources in all communities are working together and creating partnerships with available senior organizations to improve the safety and protection of seniors from financial abuse. These partnerships are necessary given the complexity of financial abuse cases and the consequences that may arise.

Increasing the presence and accessibility to community resources for addressing senior financial abuse and other types of abuse across the United States is critical. With the rapidly aging population, there needs to be more funds directed toward senior services especially in rural and high-aging density areas. Anytime a major pandemic occurs, it uncovers new needs and innovations to address those needs. Agencies and organizations need to consider the benefit that technology innovations such as telehealth platforms may have on increasing the visibility of seniors and accessibility to senior resources such as MDTs, E-MDTs, or other groups that can help address financial abuse cases and provide remote services. Moreover, additional federal, state, and local community funding is needed to support innovative approaches and network development aimed at creating communities in which seniors are safe from financial crimes and the consequences.

Appendix A: Federal Agencies

Consumer Financial Protection Bureau Consumer Financial Protection Bureau is a government agency that combines multiple services to focus on providing protection to consumers, including seniors by enforcing mandatory reporting, accountability, and federal financial laws on banks, lenders, and other financial companies to ensure fair treatment of seniors. CFPB provides resources to caregivers, service providers, and consumers to prevent fraud and financial abuse. CFPB takes legal action against unlawful practices of companies and aims to protect consumers from delivery of poor quality and services by *unfair*, *deceptive*, and *abusive practices.*

https://www.consumerfinance.gov/practitioner-resources/resources-for-older-adults/protecting-against-fraud/

1-855-411-2372 (TTY/TTD: 1-855-729-2372)

Federal Trade Commission The Federal Trade Commission (FTC) is the nation's consumer protection agency that takes legal action to ensure privacy of financial and online security by providing resources for online security, identity theft, and targeting marketers to stop unsolicited email and mail, as well as phone calls (National Do Not Call Registry is a free resource to stop unsolicited telemarketing calls).

- Privacy, Identity, and Online Security

https://www.consumer.ftc.gov/topics/privacy-identity-online-security

- National Do Not Call Registry

  https://www.donotcall.gov
  1-888-382-1222 (TTY: 1-866-290-4236)

- Unwanted Email and Mail

  https://www.consumer.ftc.gov/articles/0262-stopping-unsolicited-mail-phone-calls-and-email

Federal Bureau of Investigation (FBI) The US Department of Justice Federal Bureau of Investigation Victim Services Division (VSD) works in conjunction with a FBI victim specialist, FBI agent, and an employee from the US Attorney's Office to ensure investigation of financial exploitation and crime. The VSD aims to assist with victim empowerment and justice by contending with the aftermath of the financial offence.

https://www.fbi.gov/resources/victim-services
1-202-324-3000

Elder Justice Initiative (EJI) The US Department of Justice promotes federal, state, and local resources to enhance response, investigation, and prosecutions of financial entities targeting older adults. EJI coordinates investigations and prosecutions of financial fraud to maximize recovery and obtain proper retribution for the perpetrator for older adults.

https://www.justice.gov/elderjustice/financial-exploitation
1-855-484-2846

US Postal Inspection Service Postal inspectors are federal law enforcement officers that work with the US Attorney's Office and local prosecutors to educate consumers, as well as safeguard mail by forensic investigation and conviction of criminal cases. Since 1775, this federal law enforcement agency upholds security and safety to prevent and fight against criminal endangerment, mail and identity theft, and mail and financial fraud within the US Postal System.

https://www.uspis.gov
1-877-876-4455

Social Security Administration (SSA) The Social Security Administration provides financial support and protection of personal information and financial contributions to detect and identify fraudulent behavior. https://www.ssa.gov/antifraudfacts

The Social Security Administration also assists with people that need help managing their finances via the Social Security's Representative Payment Program. This program designates a Representative Payee to an individual beneficiary who is incapable of managing or appointing the management of their Social Security and/or Supplemental Security Income (SSI). The Representative Payee appointed by the Social Security Administration must furnish the SSA with documentation of all payments and expenses exchanged.

https://www.ssa.gov/payee
1-800-772-1213 (TTY 1-800-325-0778)

Office of the Inspector General (OIG) SSA works with the lead agency for fraud detection and prevention and the Office of the Inspector General to collect stolen money and prosecute the criminals. The OIG also combines resources of the federal, state, and local law enforcement to prevent and combat Medicare Fraud.

https://oig.ssa.gov

- Medicare. Reporting Medicare Fraud.

https://www.medicare.gov/forms-help-resources/help-fight-medicare-fraud/how-report-medicare-fraud
1-800-633-4227 (TTY 1-877-486-2048)

Department of Veterans Affairs (VA) Fiduciary Program The VA's Fiduciary Program protects veterans and other beneficiaries that are incapable of managing their finances by appointing a fiduciary. The beneficiary can choose a beneficiary, either family or friend, which undergoes criminal investigation, credit report, interview, and references. If no one is available, the VA will assign a fiduciary.

www.benefits.va.gov/fiduciary
1-888-407-0144

Appendix B: Legal Services

National Eldercare Locator The Eldercare Locator is a national referral and information resource of the Administration on Aging (AoA), an agency of the US Administration for Community Living and National Association of Area Agencies on Aging (n4a). The Eldercare Locator connects state-, local-, and community-based agencies with older adults and their caregivers.

https://eldercare.acl.gov
1-800-677-1116

Legal Services Corporation (LSC) The Legal Services Corporation is a non-profit, grant-making governmental organization that provides older adults with high-quality civil legal assistance involving unlawful financial lenders, bankruptcy, and management of debt.

https://www.lsc.gov/what-legal-aid/find-legal-aid
1-202-295-1500

Fee-for-Service Lawyers. The American Bar Association's Legal Services Division provides a public service that provides resources to older adults and assists low-income, active military service members, military families, veterans, and unbiased referrals to affordable lawyers.

https://www.americanbar.org/groups/legal_services/flh-home
1-800-285-2221

Appendix C: Accounting Services

American Institute of Certified Professional Accountants (AICPAs) The American Institute of CPAs is the largest association representing the CPA profession that provides tax planning and financial education, as well as supports advancement of the financial reporting system, and identifies and prohibits financial fraud.

- Find a Certified Public Accountant

https://www.aicpa.org/forthepublic/findacpa.html

- Elder Planning and Life Transitions after Retirement

https://www.aicpa.org/interestareas/personalfinancialplanning/resources/elder-planningservices.html
1-888-777 7077

References

1. Acierno R, Hernandez MA, Amstadter AB, Resnick HS, Steve K, Muzzy W, Kilpatrick DG. Prevalence and correlates of emotional, physical, sexual, and financial abuse and potential neglect in the United States: the National Elder Mistreatment Study. Am J Public Health. 2010;100(2):292–7.
2. MetLife Mature Market Institute. The MetLife study of elder financial abuse: Cimes of occasion, desperation, and predation against America's elders. New York. 2011. Retrieved from https://www.metlife.com/assets/cao/mmi/publications/studies/2011/mmi-elder-financial-abuse.pdf. Accessed May 2020.

3. Burnett J, Jackson SL, Sinha A, Aschenbrenner AR, Xia R, Murphy KP, Diamond PM. Differential mortality across five types of substantiated elder abuse. J Elder Abuse Negl. 2016;28(2):59–75.
4. Wood S, Rakela B, Liu PJ, Navarro AE, Bernatz S, Wilber KH, Alan R, Homier D. Neuropsychological profiles of victims of financial elder exploitation at the Los Angeles County Elder Abuse Forensic Center. J Elder Abuse Negl. 2014;26(4):414–23.
5. U.S Department of Justice, Elder Justice Initiative: https://www.justice.gov/elderjustice Accessed May 2020.
6. U.S. Government Accountability Office. Elder justice: national strategy needed to effectively combat elder financial exploitation (Publication No. GAO-13-110). 2012. Retrieved from http://www.gao.gov/products/GAO-13-110. Accessed May 2020.
7. Consumer Financial Protection Bureau: https://files.consumerfinance.gov/f/documents/bcfp_fighting-elder-financial-exploitation_community-networks_report-summary.pdf. Accessed May 2020.
8. Social Security Administration. Adult protective services functions and grant programs. 2017. Retrieved From: Https://www.Ssa.Gov/Op_Home/Ssact/Title20/2042.Htm. Accessed May 2020.
9. Ramsey-Klawsnik H, Burnett, J. Adult protective services program response to self-neglect. J Elder Abuse Negl; 2020. In Press.
10. CDC. Elder abuse surveillance: uniform definitions and recommended data elements. 2016. Retrieved from: https://www.cdc.gov/violenceprevention/pdf/EA_Book_Revised_2016.pdf. Accessed May 2020.
11. Texas Human Resources Code 48.002. https://statutes.capitol.texas.gov/Docs/HR/htm/HR.48.htm. Accessed May 2020.
12. American Bar Association Commission on Law and Aging: Elder Abuse Reporting https://www.americanbar.org/content/dam/aba/administrative/law_aging/2020-elder-abuse-reporting-chart.pdf. Accessed May 2020.
13. National Adult Protective Services Organization.: https://www.napsa-now.org/. Accessed May 2020.
14. National Center on Elder Abuse.: https://ncea.acl.gov/NCEA/media/publications/APS-Flow-Chart.pdf. Accessed May 2020.
15. Jackson SL, Hafemeister TL. How do abused elderly persons and their adult protective services caseworkers view law enforcement involvement and criminal prosecution, and what impact do these views have on case processing? J Elder Abuse Neglect. 2013;25(3):254–80.
16. National Sheriffs Association of Triads: https://www.sheriffs.org/programs/national-triad. Accessed May 2020.
17. Wigglesworth A, Mosqueda L, Burnight K, Younglove T, Jeske D. Findings from an elder abuse forensic center. Gerontologist. 2006;46(2):277–83.
18. Gassoumis ZD, Navarro AE, Wilber KH. Protecting victims of elder financial exploitation: the role of an Elder Abuse Forensic Center in referring victims for conservatorship. Aging Ment Health. 2015;19(9):790–8.
19. Navarro AE, Gassoumis ZD, Wilber KH. Holding abusers accountable: an elder abuse forensic center increases criminal prosecution of financial exploitation. The Gerontologist. 2013;53:303–12.
20. National Institute of Justice Elder Abuse Multidisciplinary Team Resource page.: https://www.justice.gov/elderjustice/mdt. Accessed May 2020.
21. Older Americans Act: https://acl.gov/about-acl/authorizing-statutes/older-americans-act. Accessed May 2020.
22. National Association of Area Agencies on Aging.: https://www.n4a.org/about. Accessed May 2020.
23. Administration on Community Living Elder care locator.: www.eldercare.ac.gov. Accessed May 2020.

24. American Association of Retired Persons: https://www.aarp.org/legal-counsel-for-elderly/what-we-do/info-2017/consumer-fraud-financial-abuse.html. Accessed May 2020.
25. Better Business Bureaus: https://www.bbb.org/. Accessed May 2020.
26. Sacks D, Das D, Romanick R, Caron M, Morano C, Fahs M. The value of daily money management: an analysis of outcomes and costs. J Evid Based Soc Work. 2012;9:498–511.
27. American Association of Daily Money Management: https://secure.aadmm.com/what-is-a-dmm-pdmm/. Accessed May 2020.
28. Acierno R, Watkins J, Hernandez-Tejada MA, Muzzy W, Frook G, Steedley M, Anetzberger G. Correlates of Financial Management in the National Elder Mistreatment Stusy Wave II. J Aging Health. 2018;31(7):1196–211.
29. Office for Victims of Crime, Faith Organizations: https://www.ovc.gov/publications/bulletins/elderfraud_case/pfv.html. Accessed May 2020.
30. Senior Safe Act: https://www.govtrack.us/congress/bills/115/hr3758. Accessed May 2020.
31. National Center on Elder Abuse Guardianship Resource.: https://ncea.acl.gov/NCEA/media/Publication/NCEA_GuardianStandardsFS2017.pdf. Accessed May 2020.
32. American Bar Association Commission on Law and Aging: Legal Resources: https://www.americanbar.org/groups/law_aging/resources/. Accessed May 2020.
33. Meals on Wheels of America: https://www.mealsonwheelsamerica.org/learn-more/national. Accessed May 2020.

Chapter 12
Elder Abuse Multidisciplinary Teams

Julia Margaret Rowan, Georgia J. Anetzberger, Diana Homeier, and Gerson Galdamez

Elder abuse victims suffer emotional trauma and distress, emergency hospitalization, and higher mortality [13]. Financial abuse and neglect are the deadliest forms [9]. Financial exploitation alone costs US victims 30 billion dollars each year [22]. Societal costs include undue medical care usage, facility placement [13], and emotional duress of loved ones [7]. A myriad of elder abuse interventions aim to improve victim safety and address trauma and financial impacts. Investigations assess the nature of the abuse and risk of continued harm and help determine which remedies are appropriate (e.g., criminal justice, civil law, victim advocacy, community-based services and supports, counseling, credit repair, case management, and medical care). The numerous agencies needed for comprehensive response necessitate a team approach.

Multidisciplinary teams (MDTs) convene a variety of professionals to address abuse and are considered an essential tool [8, 28]. Each agency and discipline bring different perspectives, contributions, and measures of success. This range of perspectives is both a strength and a challenge in establishing and sustaining MDTs [3].

J. M. Rowan (✉) · G. Galdamez
Leonard Davis School of Gerontology, University of Southern California, Los Angeles, CA, USA
e-mail: wysong@usc.edu; https://gero.usc.edu/secure-old-age/; ggaldame@usc.edu

G. J. Anetzberger
Schools of Applied Social Sciences and Medicine, Case Western Reserve University, Cleveland, OH, USA
e-mail: g.anetzberger@csuohio.edu

D. Homeier
University of Southern California, Los Angeles, CA, USA
e-mail: Diana.Homeier@med.usc.edu

R. M. Factora (ed.), *Aging and Money*,
https://doi.org/10.1007/978-3-030-67565-3_12

Four decades of implementation, study, and proliferation offers guidance for those starting new teams. The purpose of this chapter is to provide an overview of MDTs, particularly for medical professionals addressing financial exploitation. Section "Multidisciplinary Teams—History and Overview" reviews a brief history, followed by MDT structures and activities. Section "Considerations for the Development of MDTs" provides content related to participating in MDTs, such as communication strategies and the developmental nature of teams. Section "Benefits, Challenges, and Measuring Success" offers a glimpse into currently known benefits and challenges, evaluation, and measuring success.

Multidisciplinary Teams—History and Overview

Origin and Diffusion of Multidisciplinary Teams

The multidisciplinary approach to elder abuse began with the earliest conceptualization of adult protective services (APS) as an intervention for self-neglect and financial exploitation. Community dialogues in places like Chicago and San Diego during the 1950s led to usually government-funded demonstration projects during the 1960s, which examined how to best structure and organize APS. Project evaluations suggested that multidisciplinary perspectives were important for problem diagnosis and case planning, but even more often for service referral and delivery, highlighting social work, medicine, psychiatry, and law as key disciplines [4].

Emergence of elder abuse as a complex problem of concern to older Americans during the 1980s cemented the need for a multidisciplinary approach, particularly following the passage of intersecting state laws with multiple implementing service systems. Sometimes borrowed from other aspects of family violence or problem areas (e.g., fatality review teams) and other times unique to elder abuse (e.g., financial abuse specialist teams ([FAST])), MDTs have emerged as a cornerstone of elder abuse work [3, 6]. They have also become increasingly numerous, diversified, and formalized over time [16, 31]. The importance of MDTs is rarely challenged, and their presence has become deeply entrenched in practice.

The number of teams nationwide has increased tenfold from 31 in 2003 to 324 [16, 31]. The importance and spread of MDTs has been bolstered by national efforts in recent years. The first was the Elder Justice Roadmap, a strategic planning resource "by the field, for the field" to address elder abuse. Funded through the US Department of Justice with support from the US Department of Health and Human Services, it lists 121 action recommendations across the 4 domains of policy, direct services, education, and research. Many high-priority recommendations deal with MDTs [10]. Since its dissemination, the Roadmap has inspired the development and expansion of elder abuse initiatives nationwide, including MDTs. The second effort was a day-long symposium held a year later in New York. It produced and nationally disseminated a report titled "Elder Abuse Multidisciplinary Teams: Planning for the Future," which contains four priorities for the field: research demonstrating the value of MDTs, more pervasive advocacy on elder justice, sustained funding for MDTs, and guidance for the startup and practice of MDTs [8]. The third effort, launched in 2016, reflects recommendations from the Roadmap and MDT symposium. The US Department of Justice's (DOJ) Elder Justice Initiative established an MDT Technical Assistance Center that offers tools, resources, and individualized consultations to facilitate the expansion of elder abuse case review MDTs across the nation. Major elements of this work include an MDT needs assessment survey, network locator map, webinars on MDTs and Center activities, an MDT guide and toolkit, and a peer support online community for MDT members and coordinators [36]. Finally, the University of Southern California's Center on Elder Mistreatment (2020) received an Administration for Community Living (ACL) grant to improve knowledge about MDTs, with a particular emphasis on elder abuse forensic centers, and to promote their implementation and replication nationally. Elements of this effort include an inventory and in-depth survey of MDTs as well as forensic center products, such as evidence of their effectiveness and information on best practices and model replication [34].

Multidisciplinary Team Variation

Teams have been anecdotally classified into two categories: general and specialized. General MDTs consider cases representing all forms of elder abuse. Accordingly, they are comprised of a broad spectrum of representatives. Specialized MDTs focus on one elder abuse form or circumstance, and team composition reflects the disciplines key to that area (Table 12.1).

Teams Addressing Financial Exploitation

All types of elder abuse MDTs can address situations involving the financial exploitation of older adults [11]. However, three teams place exclusive or primary emphasis: FAST, forensic centers, and enhanced MDTs (E-MDTs). Each has capacity for related case review and handling through targeted team composition, procedures, and/or resources. Among them, FAST was the earliest to appear, is more widespread geographically, and remains the only one to solely concentrate on financial exploitation. Created in 1993 to combat financial exploitation as a growing problem in Los Angeles, California, FAST is characterized by immediate or early response, expert consultation, and service integration. Team composition varies locally, but more than other MDT types, FAST is likely to include financial and estate planners, securities and real estate brokers, and Social Security Administration representatives [1, 6].

Due to the complexity of financial exploitation and difficulty in criminally investigating and prosecuting it, forensic center teams tend to consider more cases alleging this elder abuse form than any other. For instance, the Los Angeles Elder Abuse

Table 12.1 Types of elder abuse multidisciplinary teams (MDTs)

General MDTs
Adult protection team: Organized by a local adult protective services (APS) program, sometimes under legal mandate, to assist APS staff in case assessment and securing resources through connection and consultation with other community agencies, e.g., Illinois and Ohio are required by law to have such teams
Community case consult team: Generally under the auspice of an elder abuse network or other partnership for case review and recommendation using the perspectives and expertise of a broad range of organizations and professional disciplines, e.g., the Institute on Aging of San Francisco has a long-standing elder abuse MDT
Enhanced team: Pioneered by the New York City Elder Abuse Center and Lifespan of Rochester, to serve as a central point for professionals to work collaboratively on elder abuse cases in a given locale; using a case consultation model that emphasizes shared goals, definitions, decision-making, and partnership in problem identification and resolution for cases that involve financial exploitation and other co-occurring forms of elder abuse, e.g., New York City has a team in each of its five boroughs
Specialized MDTs
Fatality review team: Examining fatalities that may be related to elder abuse in order to prosecute individual cases as well as identify systemic problems toward promoting policies and practices that prevent future deaths; including as members those often not found on other types of MDTs, such as representatives from the coroner's office, funeral homes, and hospice agencies, e.g., the American Bar Association's Commission on Law and Aging recently identified 35 elder abuse or domestic violence fatality review teams in 13 states that conduct elder death reviews [2]
Financial abuse specialist team (FAST): Providing consultation on difficult elder financial exploitation cases, using professional partners with special expertise and practice toward comprehensive assessment and service delivery in this problem area, e.g., Orange County, California, FAST operates under the auspice of the County Council on Aging, and the Illinois FAST was developed by AgeOptions in metropolitan Chicago
Forensic center team: Attempting to apply scientific knowledge to elder abuse as a legal concern by convening professionals from diverse disciplines for case analysis, problem-solving, service planning and provision, and prosecution; using methods like victim interviews, evidence review, research, and expert consultation, e.g., evaluations of the Los Angeles Elder Abuse Forensic Center have made it the best known such center in the country, with evidence that team outcomes significantly differ from usual care with respect to increased prosecutions and conservatorships along with reduced elder abuse reoccurrence [18, 23]
Geriatric or medical assessment team: Based in a medical facility, most commonly a healthcare system; focusing on clinical evaluation, recommendation, and management of complex elder abuse cases; minimally using the expertise of physicians, nurses, and social workers, e.g., the Texas Elder Abuse and Mistreatment Team (TEAM) is located in Houston and represents a partnership of the University of Texas Health Science Center, McGovern Medical School, and Texas Department of Family and Protective Services
Hoarding team: Focusing on severe hoarding situations, many of which qualify as self-neglect under various state laws; including professional disciplines not typically found in other MDT types, such as animal control, code enforcement, and public health agents, e.g., hoarding teams are found in Cuyahoga County, Ohio, and Kalamazoo, Michigan, as well as 83 other locations in the USA, Canada, and Australia [14]

Forensic Center team finds that nearly three of four cases brought for review involve financial exploitation [23, 24]. Membership of forensic center MDTs includes client services, investigators, and the justice system toward the improved safety, protection, and service access for victims. Outcomes are thought to extend to professionals through learning and collaboration and the community at large with improved detection and prevention [40]. For these reasons, the study and replication of forensic centers was an action item in the Elder Justice Act [35].

Finally, E-MDTs place special emphasis on financial exploitation cases, with a composition of members from disciplines key to investigating, intervening, and preventing this problem as it affects older adults. These professionals include forensic accountants, neuropsychologists, geriatric psychiatrists, and community legal services providers. Like forensic centers, E-MDTs collaboratively evaluate victim cognitive abilities and develop case plans tailored to victim needs and priorities in response. Among the three financial exploitation-focused teams, enhanced teams are the most recently developed and newly identified for replication through the Office for Victims of Crime Act grant initiative [37].

Forensic centers and enhanced MDTs have many of the same processes and include expert consultants for specialized assessment and document review. Categorical distinction is unclear and may be regionally based, with the forensic center in California and E-MDTs in New York. One structural distinction in E-MDTs is the use of "hub" teams, where several E-MDTs are housed within a single organization and facilitators oversee multiple teams.

Activities and Structure

The most valued activity of elder abuse MDTs is collaborative problem-solving and expert consultation on individual cases of elder abuse. Also highly rated, and often occurring as a result of cross-agency discussions, is networking across professional groups. While formal educational presentations may be offered in most teams and were rated highly in 2003 [31], a much smaller proportion of present-day team participants consider such presentations to be the most important aspect of meeting [16]. Other activities carried out within MDTs are service gap identification, planning community education, and advocating for change [31].

Case review processes uniquely suited for investigating and responding to financial exploitation include identification of information required to assess the client, alleged perpetrator, and case facts; analysis of the situation across the themes of safety risks, financial vulnerability, and crime occurrence; and determination of case goals toward protection of the victim's safety, welfare, and assets [25]. The most robust teams utilize case discussion to determine a coordinated plan of action, with tasks delegated among team members, and ongoing communication regarding completion of tasks and the flow of documents. If needed, continued discussion and troubleshooting may occur in between or at subsequent meetings [16, 24, 40]. To support this integrative, coordinated, case "adoption" by the team [40], it is suggested meetings occur at least twice a month [16]. Among the range of teams currently in operation, 80% hold meetings 60–90 minutes long for review of 1–2 cases per meeting, with an average of 11–30 cases per year. Financial exploitation is the most common form of abuse reviewed, followed by physical abuse and neglect [16].

Formalization and Leadership Structures

Methods of formalization utilized by MDTs systematize processes and agreements among members and may include summarization of findings, use of contracts/MOU, structured case review guidelines, policy and procedure manuals, job descriptions, orientation manuals, and term limits [31]. Most MDTs require that agencies sign an MOU or MOA, outlining expectation of participation and team protocols, and consultants providing paid work to the team (e.g., forensic accountants, psychologists, attorneys) may alternatively sign a contract with similar stipulations. Sample MOUs, contracts, procedure manuals, and job descriptions are offered on the DOJ's Technical Assistance Center [36]. Decisions on MDT formalization are best determined collaboratively, weighting the preferences and needs of the core agencies whose participation is necessary for the team to function effectively. MDTs are often housed within an organization, which may offer a starting point for preferences on team operation. Such sponsoring agencies are potential sources of commitment from partnering community stakeholders and in-kind resources such as meeting space, staff to oversee MDT operation, and the participation of certain members [16]. Half of MDTs in the USA were housed within a healthcare system or organization [16], underscoring the key role that healthcare organizations offer in addressing abuse.

Dedicated staff assigned to MDT coordination and oversight is an essential ingredient in assuring coherence and maximizing capacity. Approximately half of MDTs are led by a coordinator who manages tasks related to operation, such as meeting setup (e.g., case intake and selection, meeting announcements, agenda distribution), leading meetings (e.g., assuring adherence to agenda, facilitating case discussion, taking minutes), member oversight (recruitment, establishing contracts or memoranda of understanding [MOUs], training, retention), and coordination of follow-up on case activities taken on by the team [16]. Many teams also have a leadership board for policy decisions that require deliberation across core participating agencies. The primary function of this structure is to assure that team policies honor the policies of core agencies while maximizing collaboration [39]. This is most important at the development stage, and once the team is functioning, a leadership board may facilitate agreement on adaptations of the MDT's policies, engagement of key community stakeholders, and sustainability planning. It is recommended that MDTs conducting case reviews create policies defining member roles and expectations and create agreements about information use and sharing. Sharing details and documents is often necessary to learn about the case and collaboratively discuss options, and must be protected from inappropriate use.

Membership

Member selection should be based on the activities needed to carry out the mission and specific objectives of the MDT, with considerations of individual expertise, and the authority of their agency, in contributing to the collective capacity [8]. Adult protective services (APS) are common first responders to suspicions of elder abuse and are members of all MDTs recently identified, with attendance at every meeting in 90% of MDTs. Other crucial agencies found in majority of teams are law enforcement (in 96% of teams), case management (68%), medical professions such as nurses or physician assistants (67%), community-based mental health services (65%), prosecution (63%), victim advocacy (62%), the public guardian or conservator (57%), and Area Agencies on Aging (56%) [16]. One-fifth of existing MDTs have physicians [16], who are particularly valued members that conduct physical or cognitive examinations and review medical documentation. They are positioned to serve as expert witnesses for court testimony and to assess healthcare needs or communicate with healthcare providers already involved with abuse victims [33]. Psychologists (found in 17% of teams) provide in-depth capacity assessment [15], and forensic accountants examine financial documents for fraudulent transactions [12].

Several agencies may not be as crucial to the team function but offer assistance and services to attenuate the consequences of abuse and reduce dependency on the abuser (e.g., trauma-informed therapy, caregiver respite, creditor intervention, or home-delivered meals). Formalized membership of these agencies can expedite and coordinate services along with other case plan action items. MDTs focusing on financial exploitation may also include members from various financial industries who can examine documents, recommend courses of action, and advise on industry standards and regulation [1]. It is important to weigh the benefits of a professionals' membership against challenges posed. Inclusion of individuals within private for-profit businesses requires careful management of conflict of interest and confidentiality and may hinder full participation of the core public agencies. In some cases, members representing regulatory agencies (e.g., departments of insurance or real estate, bar association) may be just as knowledgeable and more appropriate if experienced at investigating malpractice. Sometimes, additional experts or agencies not commonly associated with addressing elder abuse are sought based on the needs observed within the team. For example, some MDTs include code enforcement and animal control to assist with self-neglect, which is often concurrent with elder abuse, and general contractors who aid in identification of contractor scams. The size of the MDT and range of professionals invited must be weighed against ease of information sharing and ability to make a group decision, which are more cumbersome in a large team.

Considerations for the Development of MDTs

Teams are dynamic. Members of well-established MDTs describe a synergy in which the power of the whole exceeds the sum of constituent capabilities. There is a developmental progression that occurs once the first meeting is convened—which is often itself a major feat—and it is essential to recognize that the journey to becoming a robust team is best supported with careful attention to relational and processual aspects. Developing a team identity requires learning about the capabilities and priorities of other members and the ability to listen to disparate views [36]. This necessitates individuals to listen and learn about the realities of other agencies and professions. It may help to recognize that (1) each member has an individualized conception of what actions are appropriate based on their professional role and personal experiences and (2) those who arrive to contribute to an MDT are likely well-intentioned. Remembering these commonalities, and the overarching aim to help victims of elder abuse, aids in effective communication toward the generation of a cohesive MDT [36].

A useful framework to understand teams from a developmental perspective is Bruce W. Tuckman's descriptions of the stages "Forming, Storming, Norming, and Performing," each having distinct characteristics and value [32]. During "forming," members may experience a combination of excitement of potentiality and performance anxiety. A key aim during this stage is creating goals, developing processes, and defining roles. At this time, productivity may appear low; products of this phase are clarified expectations and trust, which together form a foundation for accomplishments to come. "Storming" is typified by disillusionment and frustration about a lack of progress toward the initial vision and may result in criticism and lashing out among members. It may be helpful for teams to reconceptualize aims and define smaller marks of progress and, in some circumstances, develop conflict management skills. During "norming," teams acknowledge their progress and value flexible expectations and member inclusivity. Comfort expressing true feelings, appreciation for alternate views, and constructive criticism are coupled with an increase in substantive productivity. This is a fertile period for initiating process and outcome evaluation. Finally, "performing" teams become attuned to problem-solving as a group and appreciate one another's differences as attributes that enhance group capability. The progression is not always linear, and identifying the stage the team is operating within can provide a basis for a conversation on how to respond to maximize progress [32]. For example, "forming" may return with changes to the internal and external environment, such as addition of new members, major adaptations incorporated to the team, or changes within sponsoring agency.

Teams in Action: A Case Study

Figure 12.1 presents a hypothetical case study demonstrating case process of a newer forensic center MDT in the "forming" stage. It was presented by an APS caseworker for assistance assuring the client's safety and protecting her assets. This

Presentation to the Team

Ms. P, age 86, lived in a beautiful home in an affluent neighborhood. She had several caregivers providing 24-hour care because, with severe memory deficits, she needed help with meals, medication management, and bathing. One of the caregivers placed a report to APS, alleging theft and isolation by Charles, her agent acting under power of attorney. Charles forbids Ms. P to leave the home or communicate with anyone. The caregivers were instructed to direct all visitors and telephone calls to him and to keep her from seeing the mail. The caregiver said Ms. P believed she was being poisoned because Charles gives her a pill during his visits that caused dizziness, confusion, and nausea. The APS caseworker attempted visits and was refused entry each time. Cross-reports to local police resulted in assignment of a detective who showed no concern and said it was not a law enforcement matter. The APS caseworker did not believe the detective was knowledgeable on elder financial exploitation or dementia and requested the MDT's in assistance accessing Ms. P to determine thelevel of danger.

Team Review

Concern for Ms. P's safety was paramount, and the team decided that quick action was needed. The APS worker wanted the district attorney to expedite a court order removing Ms. P from her home. This spurred clarification of team member roles and what each agency *could* do. The elder abuse prosecutor explained that many detectives are not knowledgeable on criminal elder abuse investigations and offered to contact the detective to give guidance. The medical professional agreed to evaluate Ms. P's physical and cognitive status, which initiated deliberation on ultimate goals. Some team members hoped that if Ms. P lacked cognitive capacity, a guardian would be appointed that day. The representative from the Office of the Public Guardian (OPG) explained that guardianship is a multi-phased process and possibly inappropriate. Further conversation on the many safety issues resulted in the OPG representative reviewing guardianship requirements and agreeing to assign an investigator, contingent on capacity determination. Law enforcement's assistance was required to assure access to Ms. P, so the prosecutor contacted the involved detective, who agreed to assist the team.

Teamwork in the Field

A home visit was conducted that same day by the APS social worker, medical professional, and detective. With the detective's assistance, the team was permitted to evaluate Ms. P, which involved an interview, medical history, review of medications, vital signs, and cognitive testing. Ms. P grossly underestimated the value of her home and was unclear on her net worth or monthly expenses. She asked to look through her checkbook with the examiners. Ms. P had written checks worth thousands of dollars to Charles and his family members in just the prior week and could not explain what that money was for. On cognitive testing, Ms. P exhibited impaired memory and executive function. For medication review, the caregiver provided her pill box and prescriptions. The medical professional called the primary care physician's office for verification, and it was discovered that an additional prescription, a benzodiazepine, was prescribed per Charles' request and likely the pill given by Charles. The medical professional completed a capacity declaration and forwarded it to the OPG representative. The detective documented the checks and her vulnerability, which was explained by the medical professional. He agreed to begin an elder financial abuse investigation.

Results of Multidisciplinary Team Intervention

One week later, the team reviewed the actions. A guardianship referral was placed, and the following OPG investigation found a nephew who had been trying, unsuccessfully, to communicate with Ms. P. He was interested in acting as her guardian but did not know how to proceed. The OPG educated him about the responsibilities and process of guardianship, and within 2 weeks, her nephew was appointed guardian and fired Charles. Ms. P's caregivers remained, which allowed her to continue living in her own home. Several months later, the district attorney filed an elder abuse charge against Charles, resulting in a successful prosecution.

Fig. 12.1 Case study: a team in action

case study demonstrates "forming," evident by team member's limited awareness of the extent of other members' role and the process and capability of their agencies. While some of this knowledge can be, and often is, offered in member onboarding and training prior to team participation, most teams rely on case discussions during meetings and collaborative fieldwork to truly understand one another and how to best collaborate. This case exemplifies that even with unrealistic initial expectations, requests and clarification, then focusing on feasible actions, produce solutions that would not have otherwise been available.

Other Multidisciplinary Groups

Multidisciplinary teams represent just one means by which different disciplines, organizations, and systems come together to better address elder abuse. Other groups are interdisciplinary teams, networks, and task forces (Table 12.2). Although all four groups differ in purpose and membership, and typically in auspice and duration as well, they have in common three characteristics: (1) belief that elder abuse understanding and response requires comprehensive knowledge and collective action and that one perspective and force is insufficient; (2) realization that elder abuse requires structures and supports which endure, with the nimbleness to

Table 12.2 Other multidisciplinary groups addressing elder abuse

Interdisciplinary teams: These teams are created by a single organization, such as a social service agency, to clinically assess and intervene in elder abuse cases handled by that organization. They tend to be composed of the disciplines represented among staff within the organization and only occasionally others outside it, such as when certain perspectives or skills are required for holistic case review or intervention and they are only available in the larger community through consultation. Lifespan of Rochester has the interdisciplinary team to coordinate services for elder abuse and other cases that cross programs due to their complexity and needs
Networks: Also called coalitions or councils, networks represent a community, region, or state in identifying and taking action to effect issues or gaps in elder abuse awareness, policy, and practice. They tend to be composed of community planners, agency leaders, policy makers, advocates, government officials, and media representatives. The California Elder Abuse Coalition and Maine Council for Elder Abuse Prevention represent state elder abuse networks. The federal Consumer Financial Protection Bureau [11] conducted research nationwide on elder abuse networks, interviewing representatives from 23 of them, discovering only 6% that specialized in preventing and responding to financial exploitation
Task forces: Also called summits and assemblies, these efforts are formed for the expressed purpose of developing a set of recommendations to address elder abuse through multisystem intervention targeting a particular geographic area or intervention approach. Often convened by a government department or official, task forces tend to be time-limited and composed of leadership from organizations charged with elder abuse work and other key stakeholders. A 50-state survey yielded 20 that had convened state-level task forces, including Arkansas and Colorado [5]

react appropriate to whatever situation is at hand; and (3) commitment to find the means for working together, no matter individual or group differences or concerns [8, 11].

The distinctions and relations among elder abuse multidisciplinary groups can change over time. More specifically, an agency that has an interdisciplinary team also can join an MDT and network. For instance, Cleveland, Ohio's Benjamin Rose Institute on Aging established an interdisciplinary team (Elder Abuse and Ethics Case Consult Team) while also engaged with a community network (Consortium Against Adult Abuse) and its MDT (Clinical Consultation Committee). Similarly, a task force can evolve into or undertake other elder abuse multidisciplinary groups. For example, Lifespan of Rochester convened a New York State summit on elder abuse during the early 2000s. The summit later evolved into the New York State Coalition on Elder Abuse, which has overseen the development of enhanced teams in upstate New York [5]. There are countless other examples across the nation of multidisciplinary groups forming, learning, and spanning into other projects. When developing an MDT, it is worth contacting other local elder abuse multidisciplinary groups, existing or expired, as a foundation.

Benefits, Challenges, and Measuring Success

Benefits and Victim Outcomes

Perceived success and effectiveness of MDTs tend to be high among members [40], and many feel they personally contribute to improved victim safety, support of client self-determination, and physical and mental health of the victim. MDTs are also perceived by members to enable person-centered outcomes: client wishes are part of the case decision-making process, and if such wishes contradict the case plan, adjustments are made. Other evidenced value of MDTs is improved ability to accomplish case goals such as prosecution and conservatorship [18, 23]. Beyond case outcomes, members experience improved capability in their work or practice outside the team and improved relationships with other professional agencies [16, 40]. The potential impacts of improving the manner in which individuals think and collaborate, and the creation of communication pathways bridging siloed systems, are difficult to quantify yet should not be overlooked in assessing the value of MDTs.

Challenges Faced by Multidisciplinary Teams

Multidisciplinary teams encounter challenges in every phase of their existence, but particularly during development and sustainability. During MDT development, these may include lack of participation by key disciplines or systems, insufficient confidence in another's intervention approach, problems in communication because of language differences, and concerns about client confidentiality and conflict of interest. Later, as MDTs face sustainability, other challenges can emerge, most commonly inadequate funding or insufficient time [17]. Of particular concern can be the declining interest and involvement of members, evidenced by absenteeism, fewer case referrals, or general disengagement, originating from increased job demands among members, oversaturation of MDTs locally, or feelings that time spent on MDT activities is wasted. Suggestions for addressing these and other MDT challenges can be found in Chap. 9 of the US Department of Justice MDT Guide and Toolkit [36].

Exploring solutions to enrolling members, and sustaining participation, can be gleaned through the perspectives of professionals who are engaged and committed to an MDT. Membership pathways vary. Many become aware of their MDT through their job or organization, and in some cases, it may be required as a responsibility of their professional role, such as APS caseworkers. Others are motivated by desire for professional input on cases. Over half join for networking opportunities, and approximately one quarter had no experience in elder abuse work prior to participation [16]. Strategies for eliciting participation should be informed by the benefits resulting from their work with the team, namely, applied learning and improved resourcefulness. This could include demonstrating to agency supervisors that MDT participation results in heightened professional acuity and productivity of their employees, such that attendance may benefit the agency overall. Once members have experienced the value of the MDT first hand, their motivation to stay is the gratification of participation, and a comparable majority view their MDT as sustainable through leadership change, stating they would continue to attend [16], suggesting that member retention may rely upon assuring their needs are met.

Complexity of Evaluating MDTs

Several published evaluations of MDTs indicate effectiveness in completion of various team goals or outputs such as conservatorship and prosecution [18, 23] and change in elder abuse mistreatment status [29]. There have been many calls for more evidence on the efficacy of elder abuse interventions and MDTs specifically [8, 10]. While it is crucial to assure accountability of MDTs in improving victim outcomes, it is unclear if experimental methods alone are appropriate or feasible to definitive testing whether multidisciplinary approaches are effective at addressing elder abuse [8, 19, 26]. There are many reasons, with two that are most relevant to this discussion. First, MDTs vary widely on a multitude of factors, some of which are difficult, if not impossible, to measure (e.g., interpersonal tension, biases). Second, MDTs are developmental social systems—and the development may be nonlinear [39]. As such, sole reliance on experimental, quantitative methods may miss nuanced causal mechanisms and may offer findings conditional upon unseen variables [30].

We have observed that the act of undergoing formal evaluation will change the way MDT members think about, and approach, their work and therefore encourage partnership with researchers and learning institutions to create MDTs with evaluative cultures. Ethnographic approaches that include observation, identification of trends, and process may be more helpful than beginning with hypotheses. The study of process is just as essential as the study of outcomes in complex social systems, so instead of asking "Does this MDT work?", we suggest, "What works, for whom, in what circumstances, and why?" [27]. Mixed methods of research, incorporation of short- and long-term feedback loops, and participatory methods would aid in the understanding of the various pathways to, and ways of measuring, success [38].

To this point, it is essential to keep in mind that there is no agreed-upon definition of success in elder abuse, nor of what MDTs are supposed to do. Although it may seem intuitive that success in elder abuse is improved safety, and MDTs are supposed to increase capability to protect older adults, the reality is murky and obscure. For instance, conservatorship and prosecution appear as major successes, unless these interventions cause disruptive changes or undesired trade-offs in the victim's life [20, 21]. The voice of older people and their caregivers is nearly absent from program planning, and little concerted progress had been made to remedy this omission [10]. However, MDTs have the greatest potential to make strides on incorporating victim perspectives, because they are predicated on multiple perspectives. No published research discusses which approaches elder abuse victims prefer and what factors should be included in measuring success. Yet, MDT participants in three quarters of the teams identified across the USA list person-centered outcomes as priorities [39], indicating that a dialogue on this topic is underway.

Final Thoughts

MDTs are a promising intervention approach in remediating elder abuse. They promote cross-organizational learning and collaboration, reduce siloed service sectors, and develop critical thinking and communication skills among participants. These teams are an important tool in investigating financial abuse, and healthcare professionals and healthcare organizations have a crucial role. Whether as leaders of teams, members, or sponsoring organizations, medical expertise is needed to support investigations and provide recommendations related to victim health. We encourage the recognition that engaging in the process of team development is just as important as attention to outcomes. It is difficult to determine an appropriate outcome, so a preceding step is to put processes in place and assess their impact. The benefits are bidirectional. MDTs provide education on elder abuse and skill development in collaborative communication. Healthcare organizations are positioned to participate by recognizing signs of elder abuse in patients and contribute to emotional and physical healing of victims.

References

1. Allen J. Financial abuse of elders and dependent adults: the FAST (financial abuse specialist team) approach. J Elder Abuse Negl. 2000;12(2):85–91.
2. American Bar Association, Commission on Law and Aging. Elder/adult abuse fatality review teams webpage: teams inventory. 2019. Retrieved from https://www.amercianbar.org/groups/law_aging/resources/elder-abuse/elder-abuse-fatality-review-team-projects-and-resources
3. Anetzberger GJ. Elder abuse multidisciplinary teams. In: Dong X, editor. Elder abuse: research, practice and policy. Cham: Springer International Publishing; 2017. p. 417–32.
4. Anetzberger GJ. The evolution of a multidisciplinary response to elder abuse. Marq Elder's Advis. 2011;13(1):107–28.
5. Anetzberger GJ, Balaswamy S. Elder abuse awareness: the role of state summits. J Elder Abuse Negl. 2010;22(1–2):180–90.
6. Aziz SJ. Los Angeles county financial abuse specialist team: a model for collaboration. J Elder Abuse Negl. 2000;12(2):79–83.
7. Breckman R, Burnes D, Ross S, Marshall P, Suitor J, Lachs M, et al. When helping hurts: nonabusing family, friends, and neighbors in the lives of elder mistreatment victims. The Gerontologist. 2017;58(4):719–23.
8. Breckman R, Callahan J, Solomon J. Elder abuse multidisciplinary teams: planning for the future. New York: New York City Elder Abuse Center, Brookdale Center for Healthy Aging; The Harry and Jeanette Weinberg Center for Elder Abuse Prevention; 2015.
9. Burnett J, Jackson S, Sinha A, Aschenbrenner A, Murphy K, Xia R, et al. Five-year all-cause mortality rates across five categories of substantiated elder abuse occurring in the community. J Elder Abuse Negl. 2016;28(2):59–75.
10. Connolly MT, Brandl B, Breckman R. The elder justice roadmap: a stakeholder initiative to respond to an emerging health, justice, financial and social crisis. Washington DC: US Department of Justice and US Department of Health and Human Services; 2014.
11. Consumer Financial Protection Bureau. Report and recommendations: fighting elder financial exploitation through community networks. Washington, DC: Consumer Financial Protection Bureau; 2016.
12. Dauenhauer D, Heffernan K, Webber K, Smoker K, Caccamise P, Granata A. Utilization of a forensic accountant to investigate financial exploitation of older adults. J Adult Prot. 2020;22(3):141–52.
13. Dong X. Elder abuse: systematic review and implications for practice. J Am Geriatr Soc. 2015;63(6):1214–38.
14. Evidence Exchange Network for Mental Health and Addictions. What are effective interventions for hoarding? 2016. Retrieved from https://www.eenet.ca/resource/what-are-effective-interventions-hoarding-0
15. Falk E, Landsverk E, Mosqueda L, Olsen B, Schneider D, Bernatz S, et al. Geriatricians and psychologists: essential ingredients in the evaluation of elder abuse and neglect. J Elder Abuse Negl. 2010;22(3–4):281–90.
16. Galdamez G. Developing a better understanding of elder abuse multidisciplinary teams: addressing gaps for research, policy, and practice [PhD]. University of Southern California; 2020.
17. Galdamez G, Avent E, Rowan J, et al. Elder abuse multidisciplinary teams and networks: understanding national intervention approaches. Innov Aging. 2018;2(Suppl 1):763.
18. Gassoumis ZD, Navarro AE, Wilber KH. Protecting victims of elder financial exploitation: the role of an elder abuse forensic center in referring victims for conservatorship. Aging Ment Health. 2015;19(9):790–8.
19. Greenhalgh T, Papoutsi C. Studying complexity in health services research: desperately seeking an overdue paradigm shift. BMC Med. 2018;95(16):1–6.
20. Lachs M, Williams C, O'Brien S, Pillemer K. Adult protective service use and nursing home placement. The Gerontologist. 2002;42(6):734–9.

21. Mallers M, Claver M, Lares L. Perceived control in the lives of older adults: the influence of Langer and Rodin's work on gerontological theory, policy, and practice. The Gerontologist. 2013;54(1):67–74.
22. MetLife. Study of elder financial abuse: crimes of occasion, desperation, and predation against America's elders. 2011.
23. Navarro AE, Gassoumis ZD, Wilber KH. Holding abusers accountable: an elder abuse forensic center increases criminal prosecution of financial exploitation. The Gerontologist. 2013;53(2):303–12.
24. Navarro AE, Wilber KH, Yonashiro JY, Homeier DC. Do we really need another meeting? Lessons from the Los Angeles County Elder Abuse Forensic Center. The Gerontologist. 2010;50:702–11.
25. Navarro AE, Wysong J, DeLiema M, Schwartz EL, Nichol MB, Wilber KH. Inside the black box: the case review process of an elder abuse forensic center. The Gerontologist. 2016;56:772–81.
26. Olsen L, Aisner D, McGinnis M. The Learning Healthcare System: Workshop Summary. The Learning Healthcare System. Washington, DC 20001: National Academies Press; 2006.
27. Pawson R. The science of evaluation: a realist manifesto. SAGE; 2013.
28. Pillemer K, Burnes D, Riffin C, Lachs M. Elder abuse: global situation, risk factors, and prevention strategies. The Gerontologist. 2016;56(Suppl 2):S194–205.
29. Rizzo VM, Burnes D, Chalfy A. A systematic evaluation of a multidisciplinary social work–lawyer elder mistreatment intervention model. J Elder Abuse Negl. 2015;27(1):1–18.
30. Smyth K, Schorr L. A lot to lose: a call to rethink what constitutes "evidence" in finding social interventions that work [Internet]. John F. Kennedy School of Government, Harvard University; 2009 [cited 2 November 2020]. Available from: http://www.hks.harvard.edu/socpol/publications_main.html.
31. Teaster P, Nerenberg L, Stansbury K. A national look at elder abuse multidisciplinary teams. J Elder Abuse Negl. 2003;15(3–4):91–107.
32. Tuckman B. Developmental sequence in small groups. Psychol Bull. 1965;63(6):384–99.
33. Twomey M, Weber C. Health professionals' roles and relationships with other agencies. Clin Geriatr Med. 2014;30(4):881–95.
34. University of Southern California, Center on Elder Mistreatment. Elder abuse multidisciplinary team project. 2020. Retrieved from https://eldermistreatment.usc.edu/elder-abuse-mdt-project.
35. US Elder Justice Act [EJA], 2010.
36. US Department of Justice, Elder Justice Initiative. Multidisciplinary teams. 2020. Retrieved from https://www.justice.gov/elderjustice/mdt.
37. US Department of Justice, Office for Victims of Crime. FY2019 competitive grant solicitation: transforming America's response to elder abuse: enhanced multidisciplinary teams for older adults of abuse and financial exploitation. 2019. Retrieved from https://www.ovc.gov/grants/pdfxt/FY2019-CompetitiveSolicitation-EMDT.pdf.
38. Walton M. Applying complexity theory: a review to inform evaluation design. Eval Program Plann. 2015;45:119–26.
39. Wilber K, Gassoumis Z, Rowan J, Galdamez G, Avent, E, et al. Final report. Developing a better understanding of a unique MDT model: the Elder Abuse Forensic Center. ACL. Submission pending. No.90EJIG0006-01-00.
40. Yonashiro-Cho J, Rowan J, Gassoumis Z, Gironda M, Wilber K. Toward a better understanding of the elder abuse forensic center model: comparing and contrasting four programs in California. J Elder Abuse Negl. 2019;31(4–5):402–23.

Chapter 13
Public Policy and Advocacy

Jennifer Drost

"HAVE HOPE"
Mickey Rooney, Senate Special Committee on Aging Testimony
March 2, 2011

Historical Perspective of US Policy

The complexity of financial abuse and exploitation of older adults in the United States are challenging to define, as are the prevention, identification, and prosecution of those who take advantage of the aged. Dramatic cases of older Americans losing lifesavings through a single scam are easily identified, quickly enraging the community and politicians. However, subtle cases of exploitation, in which money and resources are misused over time, are more difficult to recognize and complicated by undue influence and exploitation of emotional ties. For most of its advocacy history, the federal government has failed to provide consistent leadership on elder abuse. As such, local and state governments and agencies have developed independent programs. Thus, policy attempts to address this issue, and elder abuse in general, have evolved in a patchwork, piecemeal fashion. This variance resulted in disparities in response and reinforced inequities, including the morbidity and mortality associated with the financial exploitation of an already vulnerable population [1].

The history of social supports for older adults stems largely from the Great Depression, but only recently has financial exploitation been specifically addressed. Prior to the Depression, family duty prevailed in caring for the aged. Many states required families to provide for the needs of dependent older adults. As families

J. Drost (✉)
Division of Geriatric Medicine, Summa Health System, Akron, OH, USA
e-mail: DrostJ@SummaHealth.org

R. M. Factora (ed.), *Aging and Money*,
https://doi.org/10.1007/978-3-030-67565-3_13

struggled through the Great Depression, however, this changed. States began funding Old Age Assistance programs to alleviate some of the burden [2, 3]. The Social Security Act (SSA) of 1935 was one of the first efforts of the federal government to establish a safety net for those over the age of 65 by supporting established state programs [3]. Amendments to the SSA enhanced federal efforts for social security and protective services, without providing guidance on social determinants of health including elder abuse and financial exploitation. The 1961 White House Conference on Aging recommendations focused on the maintenance of financial, social, and physical independence for older adults. However, it failed to broach the topic of elder abuse [2]. While the conference stated that older adults have the right to obtain "financial support of one's family," it acknowledged that families could not be held legally responsible to provide economic support for a parent. This created the obligation for governments to protect older adults from abuses and complications of poverty [2]. The conference, though well intentioned, had no clear action plan to address issues of abuse.

Building upon these recommendations, the 1962 Public Welfare Amendment (PWA), Title XVI of SSA, authorized the creation of agencies for protective social services for aged, blind, and disabled Americans but failed to recognize the occurrence of abuse in older adults [4]. Subsequent funding was granted through Title XX of SSA, passed in 1974, for Adult Protective Services (APS) through Social Services Block Grants [1, 3].

The Older Americans Act (OAA) of 1965 and subsequent emendations continued to expand community social services for older adults. It authorized the creation of the Administration on Aging (AoA), now the Administration on Community Living (ACL) [5, 6], within the US Department of Health and Human Services (DHHS). The goal of the AoA/ACL was to support independence and community living through a network of comprehensive and cost-effective services by establishing the Area Agencies on Aging [5, 7–9]. Yet, this "age-specific" bill had only a limited segment on elder abuse, neglect, and exploitation [8]. Passed in 1992, the Vulnerable Elder Rights Protection, Title VII, addressed financial abuse and exploitation in older adults for the first time [8, 10]. Title VII required each state to establish a state legal assistance developer to increase older adults' understanding of their legal and financial rights. While significantly underfunded, it authorized $5 million in grant funding to states for public awareness and education [5, 10].

During the 1980s, congressional hearings on elder abuse, neglect, and exploitation increased. A joint hearing of the US Senate and House Committees on Aging in 1980 concluded "Elder abuse is far from an isolated and localized problem involving only a few frail elderly and their pathologic offspring. The problem is a full-scale national problem which exists with a frequency which few have dared to imagine" [11]. This concern prompted the introduction of several legislative actions including the Prevention, Identification, and Treatment of Adult Abuse Act of 1980 and the Prevention, Identification, and Treatment of Elder Abuse Act of 1985 [12, 13]. These bills, if enacted, would have further developed APS and more specifically addressed financial exploitation [14]. However, despite increased public and congressional awareness of the exploitation of older adults, political pressures to reduce the federal government's role in financing social services prevented this bill and others from passing [14]. The Elder Abuse Act did provide the first national definition of financial exploitation: "the willful deprivation by a caretaker of goods or services which are necessary to avoid physical harm, mental anguish, or mental illness" [14].

A more favorable congressional environment for social services evolved in the 1990s. Amendments to the OAA in 1992 permanently created the National Center for Elder Abuse (NCEA) housed within the US Administration on Aging [15]. This consortium of six agencies included [14, 15]:

- The National Center of State Units on Aging
- The National Committee for the Prevention of Elder Abuse
- The National Association of Adult Protective Services
- The American Bar Association Commission on Law and Aging
- The Clearinghouse on Abuse and Neglect of the Elderly at the University of Delaware

The mission of the NCEA is "to improve the national response to elder abuse, neglect, and exploitation by gathering, housing, disseminating, and stimulating innovative, validated methods of practice, education, research, and policy" [16]. The agency acts as a resource for policy makers, social and healthcare services, justice system, families, and advocates who provide care for the elderly [16].

In 2000, Congress mandated reporting the nature and extent of financial exploitation of older persons through DHHS working in consultation with the Departments of Treasury and Justice, state attorneys general, and tribal prosecutors [17]. The report, published in 2009, focused on financial abuse in the community by family or caregivers and acknowledged that there were few measures in place to protect older adults from abuse by powers of attorney or guardians [17]. The report addressed several system-related issues. These included the difficulty in determining whether financial abuse has occurred, limited resources to prosecute and remediate perpetrators, and limits in the knowledge for the effectiveness of civil or criminal remedies.

The Elder Justice Act (EJA), initially introduced into the Senate in 2003 as an amendment to the SSA, passed in 2010 as part of the Patient Protection and Affordable Care Act (PPACA) [18, 19]. After nearly 50 years of efforts, this is the first federal legislation specific to elder abuse. The legislation recognized the dearth of data regarding the scope and nature of elder abuse, neglect, and exploitation. It also identified the lack of federal oversight as a contributing factor to state funding disparities [19]. The EJA defined the complexity of the issue by stating that financial exploitation is "the fraudulent or otherwise illegal, unauthorized, or improper act or process of an individual, including a caregiver or fiduciary, that uses the resources of an elder for monetary or personal benefit, profit, or gain, or that results in depriving an elder of rightful access to, or use of, benefits, resources, belongings, or assets" [19]. The EJA authorized funding for training, services, and prevention/

intervention demonstration programs. It required the ACL to create two new advisory councils: the Elder Justice Coordinating Council and the citizen-based National Advisory Board on Elder Abuse, Neglect, and Exploitation. The Coordinating Council was charged to issue reports and recommendations to DHHS for coordination of activities as they pertain to abuse, neglect, and exploitation and to provide legislative recommendations to congressional committees [5, 18, 20]. The National Advisory Board was charged to develop strategic plans in the field of elder justice [18, 19]. While the Coordinating Council has convened several times, the Advisory Board had yet to be established in 2019 [21].

Amending earlier elder justice provisions in Title XX of the SSA, renamed *Block Grants to States for Social Services and Elder Justice*, the EJA authorized dedicated funding for specific training programs within state and local governments to combat elder abuse and financial exploitation [5, 18]. In total, $777 million was authorized for the 4-year period of 2011–2014 [18]. For the first time, Congress approved federal funding, $100 million per year, for state and local Adult Protective Services (APS) agencies. Previously, funding varied between states [3, 18]. Other funds are directed toward areas related to elder abuse, such as research, best practices, forensic techniques, and specialized centers [18].

While the EJA addressed the evaluation, interventions, and prevention of elder abuse in DHHS, it failed to include a criminal justice response through the Department of Justice (DOJ) [22]. Thus, the EJA did not achieve full integration of public health, social services, and criminal justice system envisioned. Another key limitation, the EJA offered few specifics toward the protection, investigation, and prosecution specific to financial abuse. It is important to note that implementation of these programs and activities has been limited as funding has yet to be fully appropriated due to the lack of federal discretionary spending [5, 22] (Fig. 13.1).

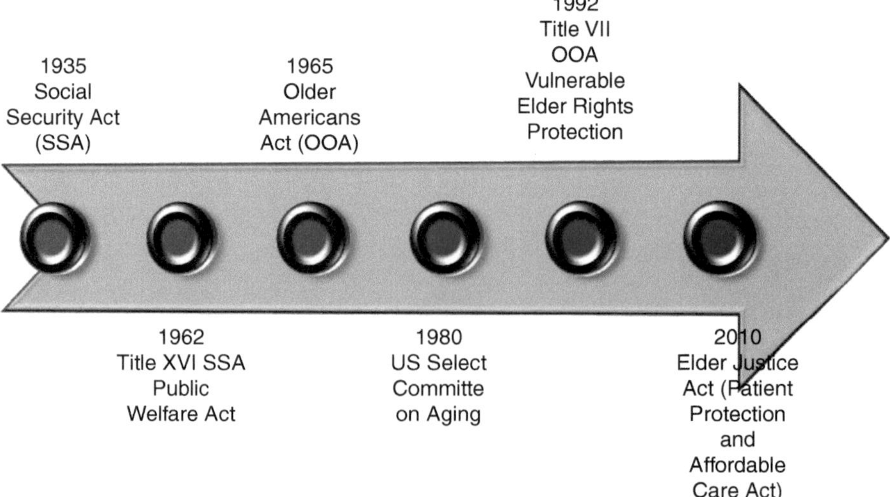

Fig. 13.1 Landmark US federal legislation addressing social services for older adults

Current Policy Initiatives

Elder Justice Act Reauthorization was introduced in the US House in each of the last three Congresses. However, reauthorization along with numerous other legislative attempts to expand the protection for older adults has failed to pass. Multiple agencies continue to advocate at the national level for elder justice reform. Most recently, the Stamp Out Elder Abuse Act of 2019 was introduced in both the US Senate and House in June 2019 [23]. That month, Robert Blancato, National Coordinator for the Elder Justice Coalition (EJC), testified before the Senate Finance Committee to advocate for dedicated funding for APS; expanding the work of the Elder Justice Coordinating Council; authority for the Advisory Board on Elder Abuse, Neglect, and Exploitation; and funding for forensic centers [21].

Reauthorization of the OAA in 2016 offered little substantive changes to previous provisions. It supports ongoing investigation into best practices for the prevention, identification, and resolution of elder abuse, neglect, and exploitation and directs the ACL to include training for service providers and increase public awareness [7]. The OAA is due for reauthorization FY 2020. Named the Dignity in Aging Act of 2019, the 5-year reauthorization would have increased funding for senior services. Though the Act passed the House unanimously in October 2019, the measure was not taken up by the Senate [24]. While services and supports have continued to operate since funding expired in 2019, reauthorization of this key legislation for senior services is vital to the continued federal response to financial exploitation of older adults.

Despite the inadequate appropriation of funds, the failure of reauthorization of EJA, and the limited success of new legislation, Congress has approved funding over the past several years for elder justice initiatives. In 2013, $2 million was provided to ACL for elder justice initiatives. Initial proposals led to the creation of the National Adult Maltreatment Reporting System (NAMRS) [25]. This reporting system was created through interagency collaboration and including multiple federal agency stakeholders (ACL, Office of the Assistant Secretary for Planning and Evaluation (ASPE), DOJ, and the CDC) and consulting expertise from NCEA and NAPSA (National APS Association) [22]. NAMRS offers the first national database on abuse and exploitation in older adults. All US states and territories are eligible to submit data, but participation is voluntary.

Federal assistance to state APS programs to investigate reports, collect and disseminate data, and develop practices was authorized under the EJA. In 2015, Congress appropriated $4 million for Elder Justice/APS. Another $8 million was appropriated in 2016 [22]. For FY 2020, the House recommended appropriations of nearly $21 million to Elder Justice/APS [26]. Funding was not matched in the Senate.

Many federal agencies hold pieces of the plan for implementation of elder justice initiatives. Justice and law enforcement, along with finance and investment regulatory agencies, continue to develop strategies independently from public health and social services. One of the biggest threats to improving the safeguards against financial exploitation in older adults is fragmentation within the federal, state, and local systems. Fragmentation of the approach can lead to duplication of services/ supports leading to further harm.

Defining a Research Agenda

A crucial limitation in the current system can be attributed to the piecemeal attempts by state and local governments to address this issue. The current approach presents many obstacles in providing effective, meaningful, and legal redress of a growing problem. Three components that continue to be echoed throughout public and scientific research are discussed below. These include defining financial abuse, reporting methods to measure scope, and setting the national research agenda [21, 27, 28].

In response to the federal EJA, states have passed more laws specific to the financial exploitation of older adults [29]. For the first time, many have defined "elder" within the law. This increased awareness, however, is paired with varying definitions and state approaches [29]. The EJA definition, although comprehensive, has its own limitations. The World Bank financial exploitation definition of "denying a victim access to or control over material goods, basic resources, and assets" is also limited [30]. Further complexity is illustrated by the NCEA, which comments that examples of financial exploitation of older adults include, but are not limited to:

> ...Cashing an elderly person's checks without authorization or permission; forging an older person's signature, misusing or stealing an older person's money or possessions; coercing or deceiving an older person into signing any document [e.g., contracts or will]; and the improper use of conservatorship, guardianship, or power of attorney. [31]

The very nature of financial exploitation causes multi-faceted confusion. Designation of abuse that includes both the act and the perpetrators' intentions complicates the identification of cases. It is difficult to recognize the difference between misconduct and mismanagement. Another example is willingly gifting one's wealth to family versus doing so secondary to undue influence. Cultural influences must also be taken into consideration.

A concise, consistent national definition of financial exploitation of older Americans is imperative. Legislative, investigative, and judiciary systems could apply a national definition universally [19]. This will allow for more effective research into risk factors, improvement in investigative strategies, and development of interventions and programs to prevent financial abuse. In addition, it will increase an understanding of the true extent of the morbidity and mortality effects of financial exploitation on aged individuals.

Investigation and prosecution into exploitative acts require complex and extended investigations and rely significantly on victim cooperation [10]. This presents its own set of complications as the victim may be the only witness to the crime and must be willing and able to provide information. Those most likely to be victims are often unable to provide a reliable history [1]. With increased federal and state supports, elder abuse forensic centers increasingly deploy multidisciplinary teams (MDTs) to investigate cases of financial exploitation. Cases evaluated by MDTs have shown increased rates of referral for prosecution and for victim support through conservatorship/guardianship [28, 32].

The National Adult Maltreatment Reporting System (NAMRS) is the first national reporting system and addresses the decade-long lack of a standardized data collection [17, 25, 33]. NAMRS collects information on agency and case components. Though reporting is voluntary, in its first year, 54 of 56 states/territories submitted data in FY 2016. In FY 2017, 55 of 56 states/territories submitted information [25]. Through building and standardizing APS programs, studying their effectiveness, and evaluating their programmatic needs and processes, the overall protective system will be strengthened [17, 33].

After establishing a national definition and reporting system, a unified research agenda can be implemented. Despite the growing awareness described, the quantity of research into elder abuse and more specifically the financial exploitation of older adults remains inadequate when compared to the scope of the problem [34]. A consistent, clear definition and hierarchy of reporting practices will ensure accurate and timely data collection and the development of accurate measures. Usage of the resultant data will spur development into specific research areas. These include the nature and cause of financial exploitation; victim risk factors, including morbidity and mortality; and perpetrator characteristics.

Forensic research can help investigators and prosecutors improve methods of securing trust with victims, as well as identification of evidence. This could lead to higher substantiation and conviction rates. Systematic evaluation of intervention and treatment methods for vulnerable older adults and alleged perpetrators will further facilitate the development of effective programs.

Professional Advocacy

Governmental agencies gather information to create programs through legislation that address financial abuse of older adults. Without sustainable funding for these programs, progress is slow at best. Given the current political landscape, it is unlikely that significant funding will be obtained in the foreseeable future. In order to move forward, grassroots advocacy efforts are needed. Assembling a comprehensive group of vested individuals is a first step. This group can work to facilitate awareness among disciplines and foster a team approach to identify and prevent financial abuse of older Americans. Interdisciplinary teams of service providers including medical personnel and financial, legal, and protective services are vital to this approach. Professions that work with older adults such as physicians, social workers, lawyers, or bankers may be involved in specific situations to recognize and report financial abuse.

Though mandatory reporting has not been shown to increase substantiation rates of claims [35], individuals should be encouraged to make reports to the appropriate state agencies if abuse is suspected. Medical professionals are often privy to patient information, including knowledge about a person's home life and vulnerabilities. Physicians, nurses, and other healthcare professionals need training to recognize risk factors for financial exploitation. These factors include dependency, cognitive impairment, depression, self-neglect, and declining health status [36, 37].

While most states have mandatory reporting of elder abuse for physicians, studies indicate that physicians make less than 3% of reports [38]. Little information exists on the recognition and reporting of financial abuse by physicians. This clearly demonstrates the need for additional education on physician awareness and understanding of financial exploitation [37]. In an Association of American Medical Colleges survey conducted in 1998, only 38% of medical schools had curriculum specific to elder abuse, with a median of one required hour of education time [39]. Of student respondents, 59% did not recall receiving education about elder abuse [39]. In Michigan, a study of primary care residency programs identified 90% of programs with curriculum in elder abuse; however, the majority of participants reported less than 5 hours of education [40].

In 2008, the American Medical Association (AMA) acknowledged the need for clinical assessment, research, and education in regard to elder mistreatment issuing a report stating:

> Addressing elder mistreatment in an aging America requires focus on increased awareness, interdisciplinary approaches, proactive physician involvement in clinical care, the education of medical students and residents, continuing education, research, and adoption of legislation. [41]

Special attention to educating current and future physicians in the face of an aging population requires collaboration. This should occur between medical schools, residency programs, continuing education, and governing bodies. Some states, such as Texas, require continuing education in elder abuse to maintain licensure [31]. This information should be included on standardized testing including the US Medical Licensing Examination, Comprehensive Osteopathic Medical Licensing Examination, and national licensing exams. Without appropriate training to identify, report, and intervene, physicians will continue to miss cases of elder abuse and leave vulnerable persons in jeopardy as financial exploitation can often be the gateway to other abuses.

Nurses are frequently the first observers to victims of financial exploitation. As primary advocates for patient care, nurses are often attuned to patient changes which may signify mistreatment [42]. As with physician training, each level of nursing education must include curricula in elder abuse, neglect, and exploitation. In 2010, the American Association of Colleges of Nursing (AACN) and the John A. Hartford Foundation Institute for Geriatric Nursing (HIGN) issued core recommendations [43].

Two of these are specific to the nursing responsibility of identification and intervention of financial exploitation. These include:

- To facilitate ethical, non-coercive decision-making by older adults and/or families/caregivers for maintaining everyday living, receiving treatment, initiating advance directives, and implementing end-of-life care
- To identify actual or potential mistreatment [physical, mental, or financial abuse and/or self-neglect] in older adults and refer appropriately [43]

Research indicates that victims of elder financial exploitation have decreased quality of life, are at higher risk for functional decline, and are three times more likely to die [1]. Therefore, these recommendations can have a tremendous positive impact on the quality of life for older adults. National nursing boards for education and licensure should be encouraged to develop comprehensive and standardized curriculum for schools of nursing and continuing education that include content on financial exploitation.

Social workers play a key role in the identification and investigation of financial exploitation. Social workers are closely involved with families and caregivers. Research indicates that the majority of financial elder abuse is perpetrated by family members [33]. This places social workers in a unique position to assess personal and family strengths as well as risk factors for financial exploitation [1, 44]. The National Association of Social Workers (NASW) practice standards recognize the ongoing need for knowledge regarding caring for the elderly and consider financial exploitation a form of family violence [44]. The standards call for the continued education of social work students and professionals to recognize the complexity of family violence and to identify risk factors and early warning signs of family violence including old adult financial abuse. Ongoing community education is also necessary to promote early intercession before abuse, whether physical, emotional, or financial, occurs [33].

Other allied health professionals, such as physical and occupational therapists, medical assistants, and emergency medical technicians, need to be aware of risk factors that may indicate financial exploitation. In 1986, the American Physical Therapy Association recognized the need for therapists to be familiar with situations where abuse may be present. The association expects therapists to educate themselves about local laws and legislation regarding reporting requirements [45, 46]. As with physicians, studies suggest many lack training and confidence to make these reports [47–49]. These allied health professionals also need standardized curricula on what constitutes financial abuse, what to be aware of, and how and where to report suspicions.

Older adults, rich or poor, are at risk for financial exploitation. Electronic banking options allow older adults to manage their financial affairs from home. Despite security safeguards in place, passwords needed to access accounts electronically can be misused or stolen outright by a family member, guardian, or power of attorney. Financial professionals [financial planners, public accountants, bankers, and crediting agencies] who are directly involved in an individual's finances can be the first to note changes in financial behaviors which may signal financial exploitation [10, 30]. In 2019, 26 US states and the District of Columbia have mandated reporting laws for financial institutions or professionals [50]. Studies have shown that banking personnel do not receive adequate training to identify warning signs and are not comfortable with reporting instances of suspected abuse [51].

Expanding programs such as the Massachusetts Bank Project on a national level could help foster education of financial experts and encourage reporting of elder financial abuse. This program, started in 1996, established collaboration between public and private entities. These included the Executive Office of Elder Affairs, the Attorney General's Office, the Massachusetts Bankers Association, the Office of Consumer Affairs and Business Regulation, and the Division of Banks [51, 52]. The collaboration provided education to participating banks and trained employees to recognize the warning signs of possible financial exploitation. The project also provided outreach to the community through pamphlets, posters, and other programs to educate older adults about the risks and methods of protection [52]. Results from the Massachusetts Bank Project suggest that bank and finance personnel are interested and willing to participate in education and skills development, with the program giving them a sense of empowerment to help older adults [51].

Early financial preparations by older adults, such as establishing financial powers of attorney or a conservator, and working with financial planners can help protect monetary assets. The Certified Senior Advisors designation is geared toward planning for older adults [53]. However, similar to family members or other trusted individuals, financial planners can turn into the "fox watching the chicken coop," thus abusing assets entrusted to them. Following through with the June 2012 call by the Consumer Financial Protection Bureau to assess the "legitimacy and authenticity of credentials held by financial planners … and looking into what sources compile publicly available information on fraudulent or misleading uses of … 'senior certifications'" would further protect older adults from financial exploitation [54]. Partnerships between the Financial Industry Regulatory Authority (FINRA) and the US Securities and Exchanges Commission (SEC) continue to expand protections for older adults. In 2013, these agencies started the National Senior Investor Initiative to evaluate practices and make recommendations regarding financial and investment supports for older adults [55]. In 2018, FINRA adopted two rules approved by the SEC. The Trusted Contact Rule (FINRA Rule 4512) requires financial advisors and brokers to make a reasonable effort to obtain contact information for a person that may be contacted if the broker/financial advisors have concerns about the management decisions of the client in the future [56]. FINRA Rule 2165 also allows for a financial advisor to place a temporary hold on accounts if financial exploitation is suspected [57].

Legal professions also need to strengthen their education and intervention strategies on abuse. Recognizing the growing issues of financial and elder abuse in the country, the American Bar Association (ABA) created the Commission on Law and Aging to help meet the legal needs of older adults and offer internships in this area to interested lawyers [10, 58]. More education is needed in more law schools. Education should include the practical aspects of drafting wills, guardianships, and other legal documents. In recent years, the National Elder Law Foundation has created a certification program to better identify lawyers who have demonstrated the knowledge and skills to provide specific services to older adults [59]. It should also include information on the challenges of psychosocial and cognitive impairment that affect many older adults. This impairment may affect their understanding and impact their ability to understand and follow through on financial advice. Teaching simple cognitive screening tools may help lawyers determine that an older client may have cognitive dysfunction that requires further assessment before proceeding with changing of a will or other financial decisions.

Law enforcement agencies as well must be armed with skills to efficiently and effectively investigate suspected cases of financial abuse. These professionals often face barriers that hinder abuse reporting and prosecution. The development of specialized teams with advanced training to investigate cases and gain the trust of the victims is essential. Improved outcomes have resulted from the creation of specialized units within state and district prosecutors' offices. The Los Angeles Elder Abuse Forensic Center is one such team which has increased referral rates to the District Attorney's Office. This leads to increased numbers of filed charges and convictions when compared to standard evaluation of cases [60]. Additional considerations to encourage cooperation include the following: victim input on appropriate punishment and restoration, video-taping victim's testimony in case of death or incapacity before trial, and allowing members of trained interdisciplinary teams to evaluate victims for cognitive impairment and financial capacity [33]. The standardization of reporting and investigating procedures combined with increased education and knowledge of law enforcement professionals is a key part in deterrence.

Self-Advocacy

Advocacy is a vital role of all who work with older Americans. Advocates are trained to recognize risk and maintain a high level of suspicion to possible exploitation. Self-advocacy is also crucial in advancing the exploitation prevention agenda. There appears to be a culture of secrecy that surrounds money matters with older Americans, many of whom are reluctant to discuss finances and financial planning even with trusted family members. As a result, exploitation is often unacknowledged. Mickey Rooney is perhaps the most well-known and widely acknowledged victim of financial violence. Reportedly victimized by his stepson, Mickey Rooney endured years of abuse, including financial exploitation. In March 2011, he spoke before the Senate Special Committee on Aging, advocating the need for federal oversight into the awareness and prevention of financial exploitation of older adults [61]. During his appearance before Congress, he stated:

> My money was taken and misused. When I asked for information, I was told that I couldn't have any of my own information. I was told it was "for my own good" and that "it was none of my business … I felt trapped, scared, used, and frustrated. But above all, I felt helpless …. [61]

Older adult victims of financial exploitation face many challenges as self-advocates. Older adults face discrimination, often viewed by others and even themselves as a burden on society. One of the biggest barriers to self-advocacy is the rationalization that financial abuse is normal and that family members or other service providers deserve the money for providing care and companionship [33]. Other obstacles to reporting include concerns about disrupting family dynamics, fear of not being believed, or that "telling" will exacerbate ongoing abuse [17]. Cognitive and physical impairments also hamper awareness and the ability for individuals to report [17]. Many older adults worry about embarrassment and that experienced exploitation will serve as proof that they cannot manage their own finances [10, 17]. Additional concerns hindering victim reporting are loss of independence, abandonment by abusers on whom they depend, and that prosecution will create further dependency [17]. Aside from the psychosocial limitations, physical constraints such as lack of transportation, chronic illness, and hearing or vision impairment also prevent victim participation as self-advocates [15].

It is important for those who are still able to tell their story to inform others of the risks and consequences of financial exploitation. All older individuals need to understand that it can happen to them. Information resources need to be readily available at sites frequented by older adults. These include senior centers, public libraries, doctor's offices, etc. In addition, information should be prominently displayed on financial and retirement websites. Once older individuals educate themselves about their risk factors, they can implement protective measures.

The Future

In the last several decades, there have been advances in legislation, societal understanding, and education on financial exploitation of older adult. These are small steps in the right direction. The economic and health consequences of elder financial abuse deserve more attention. Significant work in this area remains. Areas of focus for all entities involved with older Americans include continuing education and establishing best practices and national standards. All legislation on the financial exploitation of older Americans requires sustainable funding. In addition, such measures require the necessary clout to pursue and persecute the abusers. New legislation faces challenges in the current partisan political climate. Despite this, new bills and resolutions focusing specifically on financial exploitation of older adults continue to be introduced. One such resolution, the "Supporting the Protection of Elders Through Financial Literacy," was approved by the House in the 116th Congress (2019–2020) [62]. In addition, President Barack Obama declared on June 15, 2012, the first World Elder Abuse Awareness Day. This day focused attention on the tragedy of elder abuse, neglect, and financial exploitation of older Americans [63]. Each year, ACL in partnership with the NCEA, the National Clearinghouse on Abuse in Later Life (NCALL), the DOJ, and the University of Southern California creates and disseminates educational materials. In 2019, the theme was *Lifting Up Voices* [64]. Recurring resolutions in the US Senate affirm this priority [65]. Organizations such as the American Medical Association, the American Association of Colleges of Nursing, and the American Bar Association must continue to educate their professionals about the realities of financial exploitation. Equally important is increasing educational resources for older adults on their financial rights. This includes continued encouragement to protect themselves and knowing how to access help.

Mickey Rooney's courage to be on the front lines as a victim, to show his vulnerability, and to demand awareness, protection, and prosecution from the federal government should be an example to all victims: Even when all hope seems lost, they are not alone.

References

1. National Adult Protective Services Association. History: About Adult Protective Services from 1960 to 2000 2020 [cited 2020 January 31]. Available from: https://www.napsa-now.org/about-napsa/history/history-of-adult-protective-services/.
2. The 1961 White House Conference on Aging: Basic policy statements and recommendations. In: Senate SCoAUS, editor. 1961.
3. Social Security Administration. Social Security Online - History 2012 [cited 2020 January 10]. Available from: https://www.ssa.gov/history/index.html.
4. Cohen WJ, Ball RM. Public Welfare Amendments of 1962 and proposals or health insurance for the aged. Soc Secur Bull. 1962:3–22.
5. Dong X. Advancing the field of elder abuse: future directions and policy implications. J Am Geriatr Soc. 2012;60(11):2151–6. PubMed PMID: 23110488. PMCID: PMC3498608. Epub 2012/11/01. eng.
6. Introducing the Administration for Community Living [Text]. Department of Health and Human Services; 2012 [updated November 8, 2017; cited 2020 January 18]. Available from: http://www.hhs.gov/acl/.
7. Administration for Community Living. 2016 Older Americans Act (OAA) Reauthorization Act (P.L. 114-144).
8. O'Shaughnessy CV. Older Americans Act of 1965: programs and funding. Washington, DC: The George Washington University; 2012.
9. Older Americans Act 2017 [updated November 8, 2017; cited 2020 January 19]. Available from: https://acl.gov/about-acl/authorizing-statutes/older-americans-act.
10. Reed K. When elders lose their cents: financial abuse of the elderly. Clin Geriatr Med. 2005;21. United States.:365–82.
11. Joint Hearing US Senate and House. 1980.
12. The Prevention, Identification, and Treatment of Adult Abuse Act, H.R. 7551 (1980).

13. The Prevention, Identification and Treatment of Elder Abuse Act, (1985).
14. Quinn K, Zielke H. Elder abuse, neglect, and exploitation: policy issues. Clin Geriatr Med. 2005;21(2):449–57. PubMed PMID: 15804561. Epub 2005/04/05. eng.
15. Gorbien MJ, Eisenstein AR. Elder abuse and neglect: an overview. Clin Geriatr Med. 2005;21. United States.:279–92.
16. National Center on Elder Abuse Home 2012 [cited 2020 January 19]. Available from: http://www.ncea.aoa.gov/NCEAroot/Main_Site/Index.aspx.
17. Financial Exploitation of Older Persons: Report to Congress. In: U.S. Administration on Aging Assistant Secretary for Planning and Evaluation OoD, Aging and Long-Term Care Policy Department of Health and Human Services, editor. 2009.
18. O'Shaughnessy CV. The Elder Justice Act: addressing elder abuse, neglect, and exploitation. Washington DC: The George Washington University; 2009.
19. Elder Justice Act of 2009. In: Senate, editor. 2009.
20. Dong X, Chen R, Simon MA. Elder abuse and dementia: a review of the research and health policy. Health Aff (Millwood). 2014;33(4):642–9. PubMed PMID: 24711326. Epub 2014/04/09. eng.
21. Testimony of Robert B. Blancato, National Coordinator, Elder Justice Coalition "Promoting elder justice: a call for reform": Hearing before the Senate Finance Committee, Senate (23 July 2019).
22. Colello KJ. The Elder Justice Act: background and issues for congress. 2017.
23. Stamp Out Elder Abuse Act of 2019, (2019).
24. The Dignity in Aging Act. In: Representatives USHo, editor. 2019.
25. National Adult Maltreatment Reporting System 2019. Available from: https://acl.gov/programs/elder-justice/national-adult-maltreatment-reporting-system-namrs.
26. DeLauro. Departments of Labor, Health and Human Services, and Education, and Related Agencies Appropriations Bill. 2020.
27. Pillemer K, Connolly MT, Breckman R, Spreng N, Lachs MS. Elder mistreatment: priorities for consideration by the white house conference on aging. Gerontologist. 2015;55(2):320–7. PubMed PMID: 26035609. PMCID: PMC4542836. Epub 2015/06/04. eng.
28. U. S. Department of Justice and Department of Health and Human Services. (2014). The Elder Justice Roadmap. Washington, DC:U. S. Department of Justice and Department of Health and Human Services. Retrieved from http://ncea.acl.gov/Library/Gov_Report/docs/EJRP_Roadmap.pdf.
29. Carey C, Hodges J, Webb JK. Changes in state legislation and the impacts on elder financial fraud and exploitation. J Elder Abuse Negl. 2018;30(4):309–19. PubMed PMID: 30024309. Epub 2018/07/20. eng.
30. Price T, King PS, Dillard RL, Bulot JJ. Elder financial exploitation: implications for future policy and research in. West J Emerg Med. 2011;12(3):354–6. PubMed PMID: 21731794. PMCID: Pmc3117613. Epub 2011/07/07. eng.
31. Hall J, Karch D, Crosby A. Elder abuse surveillance: uniform definitions and recommended core data elements for use in elder abuse surveillance, version 1.0. National Center for Injury Prevention and Control, Centers for Disease Control and Prevention: Atlanta; 2016.
32. Gassoumis ZD, Navarro AE, Wilber KH. Protecting victims of elder financial exploitation: the role of an Elder Abuse Forensic Center in referring victims for conservatorship. Aging Ment Health. 2015;19(9):790–8. PubMed PMID: 25269384. Epub 2014/10/02. eng.
33. Rabiner DJ, O'Keeffe J, Brown D. Financial exploitation of older persons: challenges and opportunities to. J Aging Soc Policy. 2006;18(2):47–68. PubMed PMID: 16837401. Epub 2006/07/14. eng.
34. Corbi G, Grattagliano I, Ivshina E, Ferrara N, Solimeno Cipriano A, Campobasso CP. Elderly abuse: risk factors and nursing role. Intern Emerg Med. 2015;10(3):297–303. PubMed PMID: 25190624. Epub 2014/09/06. eng.
35. Macolini RM. Elder abuse policy: considerations in research and legislation. Behav Sci Law. 1995;13(3):349–63. PubMed PMID: 10184430. Epub 1995/07/01. eng.

36. Kemp B, Liao S. Elder financial abuse: tips for the medical director. J Am Med Dir Assoc. 2006;7. United States.:591–3.
37. Rosenblatt DE, Cho KH, Durance PW. Reporting mistreatment of older adults: the role of physicians. J Am Geriatr Soc. 1996;44(1):65–70. PubMed PMID: 8537593. Epub 1996/01/01. eng.
38. Jirik S, Sanders S. Analysis of elder abuse statutes across the United States, 2011-2012. J Gerontol Soc Work. 2014;57(5):478–97. PubMed PMID: 24811323. Epub 2014/05/09. eng.
39. Alpert EJ, Tonkin AE, Seeherman AM, Holtz HA. Family violence curricula in U.S. medical schools. Am J Prev Med. 1998;14. Netherlands.:273–82.
40. Wagenaar DB, Rosenbaum R, Page C, Herman S. Elder abuse education in residency programs: how well are we doing? Acad Med. 2009;84. United States.:611–8.
41. Report 7 of the Council on Science and Public Health: Elder Mistreatment. American Medical Association; 2008. Report No.: 429, A-07.
42. Fitzwater EL, Puchta C. Elder abuse and financial exploitation: unlawful and just plain awful! J Gerontol Nurs. 2010;36(12):3–5. PubMed PMID: 21117550. Epub 2010/12/02. eng.
43. Nursing AAoCoNTJAHFIfG. Recommended baccalaureate competencies and curricular guidelines for geriatric nursing care. September 2010.
44. National Association of Social Works. NASW Standards for Social Work Practice with Family Caregivers of Older Adults. 2010.
45. Mildenberger C, Wessman HC. Abuse and neglect of elderly persons by family members. A special communication. Phys Ther. 1986;66(4):537–9. PubMed PMID: 3960981. Epub 1986/04/01. eng.
46. American Physical Therapy Association. Code of Ethics for the Physical Therapist. HOD S06-19-47-67 ed2019 Available at: https://www.apta.org/uploadedFiles/APTAorg/About_Us/Policies/HOD/Ethics/CodeofEthics.pdf.
47. Seamon JP, Jones JS, Chun E, Krohmer JR. Identifying victims of elder abuse and neglect: a training video for prehospital personnel. Prehosp Disaster Med. 1997;12(4):269–73. PubMed PMID: 10179205. Epub 1997/09/04. eng.
48. Jones JS, Walker G, Krohmer JR. To report or not to report: emergency services response to elder abuse. Prehosp Disaster Med. 1995;10(2):96–100. PubMed PMID: 10155421. Epub 1995/03/09. eng.
49. Murphree KR, Campbell PR, Gutmann ME, Plichta SB, Nunn ME, McCann AL, et al. How well prepared are Texas dental hygienists to recognize and report elderly abuse? J Dent Educ. 2002;66(11):1274–80. PubMed PMID: 12484680. Epub 2002/12/18. eng.
50. Consumer Financial Protection Bureau. Reporting of Suspected Elder Financial Exploitation by Financial Institutions. July 2019.
51. Price G, Fox C. The Massachusetts Bank reporting project: an edge against elder financial exploitation. J Elder Abuse Negl. 1997;8(4):59–71.
52. Massachusetts Bank Reporting Project 2008 [updated 2008-05-21; cited 2020 January 18]. Available from: http://www.mass.gov/ago/consumer-resources/consumer-information/resources-for-elders/bank-reporting-project.html.
53. Certified Senior Advisor Certification and Education 2013. Available from: http://www.society-csa.com/default.aspx.
54. Consumer Financial Protection Bureau launches inquiry on elder financial abuse – Consumer Financial Protection Bureau 2012 [cited 2020 January 18]. Available from: http://www.consumerfinance.gov/pressreleases/consumer-financial-protection-bureau-launches-inquiry-on-elder-financial-abuse/.
55. Securities and Exchange Commission. National Senior Investor Initiative. A Coordinated Series of Examinations 2015.
56. Financial Industry Regulatory Authority. FINRA Rule 4512. Customer Account Information. May 8, 2019.
57. Financial Industry Regulatory Authority. FINRA Rule 2165. Financial Exploitation of Specified Adults. February 5, 2018.

58. Elder Abuse | Special Committees and Commissions 2012 [cited 2020 January 14]. Available from: http://www.americanbar.org/groups/law_aging/resources/elder_abuse.html.
59. National Elder Law Foundation. NELF fact sheet 2020 [cited 2020 February 9]. Available from: https://nelf.org/page/NELFFactSheet.
60. Navarro AE, Gassoumis ZD, Wilber KH. Holding abusers accountable: an elder abuse forensic center increases criminal. Gerontologist. 2013;53(2):303-12. PubMed PMID: 22589024. Epub 2012/05/17. Eng.
61. Testimony of Mickey Rooney: Hearing before the Senate Special Committee on Aging, Senate (2011).
62. Supporting the Protection of Elders Through Financial Literacy, (2019).
63. Presidential Proclamation -- World Elder Abuse Awareness Day, 2012 | The White House 2013. Available from: http://www.whitehouse.gov/the-press-office/2012/06/14/presidential-proclamation-world-elder-abuse-awareness-day-2012.
64. Countdown to World Elder Abuse Awareness Day 2019 [updated 4 April 2019]. Available from: https://acl.gov/news-and-events/announcements/countdown-world-elder-abuse-awareness-day-2019.
65. A resolution designating June 15, 2019, as "World Elder Abuse Awareness Day", (2019).

Chapter 14
Critical Documents Associated with Aging

An Organized Guide to Personal Files

James S. Powers, Carolyn K. Smith, Gretchen Napier, and Timothy L. Takacs

Introduction

This compendium of documents and brief explanations and definitions is meant to complement the topics discussed in this book. The list is not exhaustive, and individual circumstances differ. Consult your personal legal or financial advisor and accountant to tailor this information to individual needs.

Outline

- *Medical and Privacy Issues*
- *Caregivers, Care Managers, and Financial Concerns*
- *Legal Issues and Advance Directives: End-of-Life Care*

J. S. Powers (✉)
Center for Quality Aging, Vanderbilt University School of Medicine, Nashville, TN, USA

Tennessee Valley Geriatric Research, Education, and Clinical Center, Nashville, TN, USA
e-mail: james.powers@vanderbilt.edu

C. K. Smith
Tennessee Valley Healthcare System, Nashville, TN, USA

G. Napier
Life-Links Geriatric Care Management, Nashville, TN, USA

T. L. Takacs
Takacs McGinnis Elder Care Law, PLLC, Hendersonville, TN, USA

R. M. Factora (ed.), *Aging and Money*,
https://doi.org/10.1007/978-3-030-67565-3_14

Medical and Privacy Issues

Making a healthcare file assists families in knowing the wishes and plans of the individual. Figure 14.1 gives one example of such a form. Data provided here would contain information necessary for accessing hospitals, specialists, and other care locations to which the senior may be referred. Information needed includes medical

Name ____

Next of Kin ______________________________ Phone ( ) ____

Primary Care Provider ______________________ Phone ( ) ____

Pharmacy ______________________________ Phone ( ) ____

Allergies ____

Medical Problem	Providers you see for this (and specialty)	Providers phone	Dates you last saw provider for this issue	Dates you last saw provider for this issue	Dates you last saw provider for this issue

Surgery, Tests, Immunizations, Hospitalizations	Date	Date	Date	Date

Fig. 14.1 Example of a medical information form

Medication Name	Dosage	Reason Taken	Time(s) of Day Taken	Prescriber

Health Care Supplies and Equipment	Medical Condition	Supplier	Phone Number	Replacement date

Fig. 14.1 (continued)

history, diagnoses, medications, allergies, emergency contacts, names and phone numbers of healthcare providers, pharmacies, and health insurance information. Also included should be the names of trusted family members, attorneys-in-fact, or healthcare agents/surrogates from whom more information can be obtained when health circumstances prevent you from representing yourself.

Consumers should be familiar with terminology used when discussing healthcare coverage. The following are definitions of commonly used terms that are needed to understand how health costs are covered by government and private entities.

Medicare

- Part A: Hospital Insurance – helps pay for inpatient care in a hospital or skilled nursing facility (following a hospital stay) and some home healthcare and hospice [1].
- Part B: Medical Insurance – helps pay for doctors' services and many other medical services and supplies that are not covered by hospital insurance [1].
- Part C: Medicare Advantage – plans are available in many areas. People with Medicare Parts A and B can choose to receive all of their healthcare services through one of these provider organizations under Part C [1].
- Part D: Prescription Drug Coverage – helps pay for medications doctors prescribe for treatment [1].

Medicaid A state and federal partnership, Medicaid provides coverage for people with lower incomes, older people, people with disabilities, and some families and children [2]. Each state's Medicaid plan names and coverage vary. Coverage may include inpatient, outpatient, long-term care, home care, medications, and hospice services.

Medigap A Medicare supplement insurance, sold by private companies, can help pay some of the healthcare costs that Original Medicare doesn't cover, like copayments, coinsurance, and deductibles, and insurers selling Medigap must follow state and federal laws designated to protect you [3]. Beware of policies that sound like insurance that are not.

Dread Disease Policies Policies that pay for costs for a specific health conditions, such as certain cancers or rare chronic illnesses. They do not provide comprehensive health coverage.

Accident-Only Policies Policies that pay for costs related to an accident and not a health condition.

Supplemental Policies These could also be considered Medigap and/or cash benefits for an illness.

Discount Plans These do not provide coverage but give a discount for some services or some preferred providers. Many of these plans are fraudulent and, while using insurance language, do not in fact provide comprehensive healthcare coverage.

Stacked Policies Combinations of plans and policies sold as a bundle. These may include health insurance, dental care, death and burial policies, and disability plans.

Long-Term Care Insurance (LTCI) LTCI coverage for nursing homes, assisted living facilities, or at-home care services begins after a specified exclusion period and helps pay costs not covered by Medicare [4]. Some life insurance policies are hybrid policies permitting use of death benefits for long-term care during life and paying out the remainder to heirs at death.

Life Insurance Policy Financial pay for survivors after death, often to use for funeral and burial costs. Buy-in to this policy has a minimum requirement of investment prior to payout being available. Health conditions and cause of death may limit buy-in.

HMO Health maintenance organizations are insurance organizations which work with providers who agree to a flat fee for care instead of itemizing and billing for each individual service provided [5].

ACO Accountable care organizations are health-care networks which receive a capitated amount from Medicare to provide all healthcare services.

Below is a list of terms that define levels of care, important for understanding care needs as well as coverage benefits.

Glossary of Levels of Care

Adult Day Care structured day programs for elderly and disabled individuals permitting family caregivers time to pursue personal and employment opportunities while still maintaining affected individuals in the home setting.

Respite Care temporary in-home assistance or placement (foster medical home, nursing home, or hospital) for elderly and disabled individuals. Periods of respite, often several days to weeks, serve as breaks for caregivers.

Board and Care residence for elderly and disabled individuals who are able to ambulate or self-propel in a wheelchair. Meals, personal care, medicine administration, and group living environment are provided.

Assisted Living	residence that provides a variety of services designated to facilitate continued residence in the community for elderly and disabled persons. Assistance may include meals, administration of medication, homemaker services, transportation, health reminders, and personal care.
Nursing Home Level I (Intermediate Care)	institutional care for individuals whose functional disability requires assistance at a level of care higher than can be safely and securely provided in an assisted living facility.
Nursing Home Level II (Skilled Care)	institutional care for individuals with skilled nursing needs. Skilled care services include feeding tubes, postoperative care, wound care, and rehabilitation.

Caregivers, Care Managers, and Financial Concerns

How can family members be helpful and still preserve your dignity and independence? The following are a series of resources to be used as guidelines for issues to be addressed and options available to help understand aging and to preserve your choices.

Planning ahead is the best way to approach the future. There is a wealth of information to assist in caring for chronically ill and aging family members. Making your wishes known is the best way to ensure they will be honored. Providing knowledge of your plans provides guidance to your family.

Managing Care in the Home

Selecting who will be responsible for providing care can be a challenge. The majority of caregiving is provided by family members, but this can be stressful. Supporting the health and vitality of the caregiver is just as important as meeting the healthcare needs of the affected person.

- Remind yourself that your work has value.
- Find ways to communicate and share your needs with others.
- Consider joining a support group.
- Be organized, use calendars, and gather informative helpful resources and services.
- Nurture the positive relationships in your life with family and supportive friends.
- Give yourself a break to avoid burnout.
- Take care of your own health.
- Give yourself permission to let others assist. Make a list of how others can help: take out the garbage, go to the grocery store, unload the dishwasher, and make a meal.

It is worthwhile to determine what tasks are needed to be performed in the home before finding someone to do them. The affected elder may have certain preferences. Additionally, determining the roles of individuals and family in deciding who is and is not appropriate to bring into the home to perform these tasks is also necessary.

Caregivers are hired personnel providing personal care in the home or facility. They may also be called nursing technicians, nurse aides, sitters, non-medical in-home care providers, and private duty agencies. While there are reputable individuals who employ themselves, many work for agencies, including private duty home care agencies. When hiring an individual, it is important to recognize the employer is responsible for employment taxes, workers' compensation insurance, background checks, reference checks, etc. Professional geriatric care managers assist in coordinating services and advising families.

Care managers are often social workers, registered nurses, or other healthcare professionals with additional certification in the management of aging-related issues. A checklist of items in the Caregiving Discussion Guide (Fig. 14.2) helps to guide this discussion and helps to choose from the many available options. Issues addressed in this checklist include housing preferences, arrangements/responsibilities of caregivers, driving/transportation issues, leisure/lifestyle activities, and financial concerns.

The amount of care that an individual needs may exceed what may be able to be provided, and alternative living arrangements have to be made. Planning for this eventuality and the daily events related to relocating to a new environment are important considerations. Section 1 of the Caregiving Discussion Guide leads the family through the process of determining what an individual's preferences are regarding housing.

Often, additional assistance is needed to support keeping an individual in their current residence. Section 2 of the Caregiving Discussion Guide provides guidance on how to approach assignment of responsibilities for caregiving and arranging for such services to come to the individual's home.

Moving to a new environment could limit an individual's ability to remain active with family and in the community. Section 4 of the Caregiving Discussion Guide allows the individual to voice their preference on how they wish to continue their involvement with family and community to preserve their quality of life.

Driving is a source of independence for most people, and when this activity is restricted due to physical, sensory, or cognitive limitations, alternatives should be identified. Driving ability is a complex task that may be impaired by health conditions. There may be many reasons to consider a formal driving assessment:

- To obtain a professional opinion to verify your confidence
- To learn new strategies to keep up your driving skills in the face of illness or disability
- To consider rehabilitation
- For advice about how to meet transportation needs if driving is found to be unsafe

This document provides an outline for a discussion between an aging adult and those family and friends who are invested in that adult's wellbeing.

I. Housing
It is important to me that I remain in my home as long as possible. Should my health begin to deteriorate in a way that necessitates extra care, I am providing information as to my personal housing desires.

☐ I would like to remain in my home regardless of my condition. I would like to hire caregivers or hospice to ensure that I can remain here until my final days, regardless of expense.
☐ I am willing to move out of my home if illness/aging necessitates.
☐ I am willing to move out of my home if it becomes more cost effective to live elsewhere.
My preferred place for relocation would be:
☐ The home of a child, sibling, or other relative
☐ An assisted living facility
☐ A nursing home
☐ Other: ____

Here is what, in my mind, determines my inability to live alone in my home:

____

____

____

☐ I understand that we may disagree as to when and where relocation should occur, but I ask that you respect my wishes. There are a few exceptions where I would allow you to make the decision for me:
☐ If I lose my mental capacity and decision-making ability due to an illness like Alzheimer's or dementia.
☐ If there is a life-threatening medical emergency
☐ If I perform actions that are harmful to myself such as not taking medication, refusing to eat, or repeatedly incurring physical injuries
☐ Other: ____

Fig. 14.2 Caregiving discussion guide: values and finances

II. Caregivers

As I age, I understand that I may have certain physical and mental needs that can be best fulfilled by a caregiver. Here I am sharing my wishes as they pertain to the caregiver, should I need one.

A. Care requirements

I would like a caregiver to perform the following duties:

☐ Cook
☐ Clean
☐ Provide transportation
☐ Administer medication
☐ Bathe
☐ Other: ____

B. Care management

1. Hiring and firing

a. Before a caregiver is hired I require:
☐ A resume
☐ A background check
☐ Recommendations
☐ A personal meeting
☐ Other: ______________________________

b. The person responsible for the hiring and firing of the caregiver will be:
☐ Only myself
☐ I will take input in the hiring of a caregiver, but will be responsible for the firing
☐ I hire and fire a caregiver based on input from involved loved ones to ensure that I am receiving the best care and not being taken advantage of
☐ I am passing the responsibility of hiring and firing caregivers to:
____

2. Payment

The desired payment for the caregiver will be: $______________
The person responsible for that payment will be: ______________

Fig. 14.2 (continued)

III. Driving

I understand that as I age there may come a point when I can no longer operate a vehicle safely. Much of my independence is linked to my ability to drive, so here is what I hope will happen with respect to my driving.

A. Giving up my keys

I agree to stop driving when one of the following happens:

☐ I have an accident, minor or major
☐ I can no longer navigate
☐ I can no longer see well enough
☐ A medical professional suggests that it is no longer safe
☐ Other: ____

B. Alternate transportation

When I am no longer able to drive, I would like the following alternatives:

☐ Phone numbers provided for local senior transportation services that can take me to run errands, visit friends, or attend events
☐ An agreement with a local taxicab driver/company whom I can call and rely on when I need a ride
☐ A golf cart that I can use to drive to nearby neighbors or shopping centers
☐ Other: ____

C. My vehicle

I would like my car to be:

☐ Sold and the money used for my medical care
☐ Sold and the money used for alternative transportation
☐ Sold and the money be saved or invested
☐ Donated to a local charity
☐ Given to a relative for their personal use
☐ Other: ____

IV. Socialization/Livelihood

A. Visits/Check-ins

I would like the following interactions and provisions:

☐ Daily/weekly visits from relatives, loved ones, or senior companions
☐ Daily/weekly phone calls
☐ A person to drive me to medical appointments, the grocery store, exercise classes, or social events
☐ A person to make sure I have taken my medication and tended to health needs
☐ A hired caregiver to assist with daily physical, medical and emotional needs
☐ Other: ____

B. Socialization

It is important that I remain active and social as I age. I would like to continue my participation in/look into joining the following programs:

☐ Exercise or dance classes at local fitness, senior or community centers

Fig. 14.2 (continued)

☐ Adult day services
☐ Book clubs, card games, and other local gatherings
☐ Senior companion program, where another senior visits my home to socialize (brings me meals)
☐ Other: ____

C. Pets

☐ I plan to keep my animal companion/s as long as I am in my home, and I will be responsible for meeting all their daily needs (walking, feeding, grooming, etc.)
☐ I would like to keep my animal companion/s but I would like help with meeting their daily needs (walking, feeding, grooming, etc.)

V. Finances – attached are summary forms for all major financial information

In an effort to be prepared for financial decisions that may need to be made as I age, I am providing information regarding my personal preparations and requests.

A. Logistics

☐ I have a joint bank account for daily living expenses
The name of that person is ____________
☐ I have a power of attorney for financial matters
The name of that person is ____________
The paper document that indicates the power of attorney is located .
☐ I have a power of attorney for health matters
The name of that person is ____________
The paper document that indicates the power of attorney is located .
☐ I have a living will
That document is located ______________
☐ I have a financial planner
The name of that person is ____________
☐ I have a lawyer
The name of that person is ____________
☐ I have a health care professional to manage my care
The name of that person is ____________
☐ I have a will and/or a trust
That document is located ______________
☐ I have a safe deposit box at ____________________
☐ I have an insurance company
The name of the company is ___________
The policy is located ________________

Fig. 14.2 (continued)

B. Value statements

☐ I want all of my assets expended on my at-home care except to the point of borrowing for my care.

☐ I want to spend only my …

☐ Income

☐ Interest on my assets

☐ Other: ______________________

☐ I want all of my assets expended on my care and will borrow if necessary to maintain my standard of living and health.

☐ I am willing to borrow against my home to enable living at home.

Items I would allow purchase of with that money include …

☐ Medical supplies (such as hospital beds, wheelchairs, etc.)

☐ Medical alert system for the home

☐ Salary for a full-time/part-time caregiver

☐ Other: ______________________

☐ I want all of my assets expended on my caregiving needs to the point of selling my property and assets of pay for my care should I live outside of my personal home and at a facility. (This option will likely include qualifying for Medicaid after all assets are depleted.)

C. Bills and Routine Expenses

1. Bills

I have the following bill payments:

☐ Water

☐ Electricity

☐ Cable

☐ Phone

☐ Mortgage/rent

☐ Car note

☐ Car insurance

☐ Health insurance

☐ Credit card

☐ Home security

☐ Medical alert

☐ Subscriptions (magazine, newspaper, etc.)

☐ Other: ____

☐ I will remain responsible for all bill payments so long as I am living in my home.

☐ I would like someone to set up automatic bill pay at my bank so I don't have to worry about sending payment for water, electric, heat/air, cable, phone, etc., but I would like to retain full control of my bank account. *If automatic payments are already set up, please complete the following form "Bank Account Automatic Deposits/Withdrawals", to ensure continuity of services.*

Fig. 14.2 (continued)

☐ I would like to add a "convenience signer" to my bank account so they can help manage payments, without becoming an "owner" of the account.
☐ I would like to add another individual to my bank account so I will hold a joint account, so they can help manage payments.

2. Routine expenses
Other items I spend money on routinely:
   - ☐ Groceries
   - ☐ Medications
   - ☐ Clothing
   - ☐ Other: ____

☐ I will remain responsible for these purchases so long as I am living in my home.
☐ I would like to set up a system where I provide money for others to make these purchases for me.
☐ I would like to add another name to my bank account so they can help purchase these items.

3. Major expenses
☐ I will remain responsible for these purchases so long as I am living in my home.
☐ I would like to set up a system where I provide money for others to make these purchases for me.
☐ I would like to add a "convenience signer" to my bank account so they can help manage payments, without becoming an "owner" of the account.

D. Savings
☐ I want all of my assets expended on my at home care except to the point of emptying my savings.
☐ It is important that I maintain a percentage of my assets for my inheritors.
☐ I want all of my assets expended on my care and will borrow if necessary to maintain my standard of living and health.
☐ I am willing to borrow against my home to enable living at home.
Items I would allow purchase of with that money include …
   - ☐ Medical supplies (such as hospital beds, wheelchairs, etc.)
   - ☐ Medical alert system for the home
   - ☐ Salary for a full-time/part-time caregiver
   - ☐ Other: ______________________

Fig. 14.2 (continued)

The decision to retire from driving is difficult for many individuals. Individuals in early stages of Alzheimer's disease may benefit from a driving evaluation to determine whether they can continue to drive safely. Individuals with more advanced stages of dementia should no longer be driving. Conversation about driving should be done in a non-confrontational fashion. Section 3 of the Caregiving Discussion Guide helps outline how to approach this sensitive topic. This is a worthwhile discussion to have before a need to restrict driving arises.

The Future Caregiving Checklist (Fig. 14.3) also helps to codify plans for specific circumstances for care (including who would be present for medical emergencies, who is responsible for safety issues around the home, and arranging for backup

Medical Health Needs	**Monitor Service Providers**
Who will be responsible?	Who will be responsible?
How will it be paid for?	How will it be paid for?
What is the backup plan?	What is the backup plan?
Emergencies	**Maintain Written Records**
Who will be responsible?	Who will be responsible?
How will it be paid for?	How will it be paid for?
What is the backup plan?	What is the backup plan?
Special Treatments, adaptive equipment	**Communicate with Family Members**
Who will be responsible?	Who will be responsible?
How will it be paid for?	How will it be paid for?
What is the backup plan?	What is the backup plan?
Residential: monitoring home safety, visiting, problem-solving, annual review, recommending/managing a change in living arrangements	**Other**
Who will be responsible?	Who will be responsible?
How will it be paid for?	How will it be paid for?
What is the backup plan?	What is the backup plan?

Fig. 14.3 Future caregiving checklist

plans if the primary individual responsible is unable to deliver care). Information provided in this checklist becomes a useful reference for family members and other caregivers when unpredicted events interrupt the usual delivery of care.

Financial Concerns

Appropriate management of finances can become a source of conflict within a family. Planning for who will assume responsibilities for financial matters and disseminating this information can help to avert these problems. Section 5 of the Caregiving Discussion Guide provides a framework documenting what legal documents have been already drafted that address financial and health issues (such as durable healthcare power of attorney and wills), what individuals are already involved in portions of the financial decision-making process (executor, attorneys involved in financial matter) and may share a joint bank account with the individual for daily billing maintenance, what financial liabilities still exist (utilities, mortgages, credit card bills), and where financial assets are located (savings, pensions, etc.). Information contained in this section is particularly useful when wills are executed.

This section also allows the individual to voice how they would want their assets to be disbursed/utilized in the event that they would not be able to participate in any of the financial decision-making. Having all of this information on paper and allowing select trusted individuals access to this information would be useful in protecting against future financial exploitation.

Figure 14.4 gives an example of how to list net worth, and Fig. 14.5 gives an example of how to document assets. Figure 14.6 lists important personal documents that should be kept and suggests how long they should remain in your possession. As these documents do change over time, making sure that this information is continuously updated is also important.

A note on financial scams: the high-tech nature of banking and finance can expose seniors to fraud in very complex ways. Preventing fraud and financial identity theft of Social Security numbers and bank accounts is critical for older Americans. Monitor bank and credit card accounts and insurance benefit statements for costs that you did not incur, and act properly to correct your records. Treat insurance numbers as private and invaluable. Avoid discussion of surgery and medical procedures on social media. Older Americans are often targeted by phone calls and tend to be over-trusting of authentic sounding individuals. Remember that the Internal Revenue Service (IRS) does not notify people of tax issues by phone until it has sent written communications, usually multiple times. Consider signing up for Informed Delivery® by USPS® for daily digital scans of mail soon to arrive, to permit cross-checking for mail theft (https://informeddelivery.usps.com/).

Assets: what you own

Cash & Cash Equivalents	Total
Checking Account	
Savings Account	
Other	
Retirement Assets	
Defined Contribution Pension	
Defined Benefit Pension	
Social Security Pension	
Tax-Deferred Annuity 403(b)	
457(b)/401(k)	
Keoghs	
IRAs	
After-Tax Annuities	
Other	
Invested Assets	
Brokerage Accounts	
Stocks	
Bonds	
Real Estate Funds	
Mutual Funds	
Life Insurance Cash Value	
Other	
Personal Use Assets	
Primary Residence	
Secondary Residene(s)	
Car(s)	
Furnishings	
Jewelry	
Collectibles (art, antiques, etc.)	
Other	
Total Assets	

Liabilities: what you owe

Curr ent Liabilities	Total
Credit Card(s)	
Car Payments(s)	
Education Loan(s)	
Life Insurance Premium(s)	
Other	
Long-term Liabilities	
Primary Residence Mortgage	
Education Funding	
Secondary Residence Mortgage	
Other	
Total Liabilities	

Net worth

Total Assets	
- Total Liabilities	
= Net Worth	

Net worth calculation:
Subtract your total liabilities from your total assets to calculate your net worth.

Fig. 14.4 Summary – net worth statement *(Details contained in the following pages)*

Legal Issues and Advance Directives: End-of-Life Care

Developing an advance directive is all about personal choice, but it's also about preparing loved ones to make it easier for them to make healthcare decisions when the individual cannot. With whom is it more important to address these issues than with other family members? Receiving care that is consistent with individual values having the opportunity to make informed decisions about end-of-life care depends on the recording and sharing of these documents with families and others.

Brokerage Accounts

Broker and Brokerage Firm
Address
Contact
Phone #
Account #
Statement Location
Broker and Brokerage Firm
Address
Contact
Phone #
Account #
Statement Location
Broker and Brokerage Firm
Address
Contact
Phone #
Account #
Statement Location
Broker and Brokerage Firm
Address
Contact
Phone #
Account #
Statement Location
Broker and Brokerage Firm
Address
Contact
Phone #
Account #
Statement Location

Bank Accounts

Type of account □ Checking □ Savings □ Other
Bank Name
Address
Account #
Held Jointly with
Statement Location
Type of account □ Checking □ Savings □ Other
Bank Name
Address
Account #
Held Jointly with
Statement Location
Type of account □ Checking □ Savings □ Other
Bank Name
Address
Account #
Held Jointly with
StatemehLocation
Type of account □ Checking □ Savings □ Other
Bank Name
Address
Account #
Held Jointly with
Statement Location
Type of account □ Checking □ Savings □ Other
Bank Name
Address
Account #
Held Jointly with
Statement Location

Fig. 14.5 Your important records – ASSETS

Your Important RecordsASSETS (continued)

Retirement/Pension benefits

Employer/Type Plan
□ Defined Benefit □401(k) □403(b) □Other
Plan Administrator
Address
Phone #
Primary Beneficiary
Contingent Beaeficiary
Statement Location
Employer/Type Plan
□ Defined Benefit □401(k) □403(b) □Other
Plan Administrator
Address
Phone #
Primary Beneficiary
Contingent Beneficiary
Statement Location
Employer/Type Plan
□ Defined Benefit □401(k) □403(b) □Other
Plan Administrator
Address
Phone #
Primary Beneficiary
Contingent Beneficiary
Statement Location

Safe Deposit Box

Location	
Address	
Phone #	Box #
Key Location	
Renewal Date	
List of box contents:________________________	

Mutual Fund accounts

Name of Company/Fund
Address
Phone #
Account #
Statement Location
Name of Company/Fund
Address
Phone #
Account #
Statement Location
Name of Company/Fund
Address
Phone #
Account #
Statement Location

Annuities

Company
Contract #
Phone #
Primary Beneficiary
Contingent Beneficiary
Statement Location
Company
Contract #
Address
Phone #
Primary Beneficiary
Contingent Beneficiary
Statement Location

Fig. 14.5 (continued)

Your Important Records ASSETS (continued)

Children's accounts and trust

Child's Name
Account/Trust Type
Where Invested
Custodian/Trustee
Address
Statement Location
Child's Name
Account/Trust Type
Where Inveted
Custodian/Trustee
Address
Statement Location
Child's Name
Account/Trust Type
Where Invested
Custodian/Trustee
Address
Statement Location
Child's Name
Account/Trust Type
Where Invested
Custodian/Trustee
Address
Statement Location
Child's Name
Account/Trust Type
Where Invested
Custodian/Trustee
Address
Statement Location

Other Savings

Type
Institution
Details
Type
Institution
Details
Type
Institution
Details
Type
Institution
Details

Real Estate Owned

Address
Mortgage Amount
Title in name of
Title documents location
Insurance policy location
Address
Mortgage Amount
Title in name of
Title documents location
Insurance policy location
Address
Mortgage Amount
Title in name of
Title documents location
Insurance policy location
Address
Mortgage Amount
Title in name of
Title documents location
Insurance policy location

Fig. 14.5 (continued)

Your Important Records- ASSETS (continued)

Personal Property(Automobiles, jewelry, etc.)

Type
Make/Model
Serial/VIN#
Value
Location
Type
Make/Model
Serial/VIN#
Value
Location
Type
Make/Model
Serial/VIN#
Value
Location
Type
Make/Model
Serial/VIN#
Value
Location
Type
Make/Model
Serial/VIN#
Value
Location
Type
Make/Model
Serial/VIN#
Value
Location
Type
Make/Model
Serial/VIN#
Value
Location

Fig. 14.5 (continued)

Your Important Records – LIABILITIES

Credit Cards

Issuing Bank/Company
Name on Card
Account #
Balance
Location of Card
Location of Statement
Issuing Bank/Company
Name on Card
Account #
Balance
Location of Card
Location of Statement
Issuing Bank/Company
Name on Card
Account #
Balance
Location of Card
Location of Statement
Issuing Bank/Company
Name on Card
Account #
Balance
Location of Card
Location of Statement
Issuing Bank/Company
Name on Card
Account #
Balance
Location of Card
Location of Statement

Mortgages or Other Debts

Lender
Account #
Balance
Payment amount
Due Date
Lender
Account #
Balance
Payment amount
Due Date
Lender
Account #
Balance
Payment amount
Due Date
Lender
Account #
Balance
Payment amount
Due Date
Lender
Account #
Balance
Payment amount
Due Date
Lender
Account #
Balance
Payment amount
Due Date
Lender
Account #
Balance
Payment amount
Due Date

Fig. 14.5 (continued)

Bank Account Automatic Deposits/Withdrawals

Account Institution	**Account Institution**
Account #	Account #
Amount	Amount
Dateof Transaction	Date of Transaction
For Deposit, Received from	For Deposit, Received from
For Withdrawal, Payable to	For Withdrawal, Payable to
Account Institution	**Account Institution**
Account #	Account #
Amount	Amount
Date of Transaction	Date of Transaction
For Deposit, Received from	For Deposit, Received from
For Withdrawal, Payable to	For Withdrawal, Payable to
Account Institution	**Account Institution**
Account #	Account #
Amount	Amount
Date of Transaction	Date of Transaction
For Deposit, Received from	For Deposit, Received from
For Withdrawal, Payable to	For Withdrawal, Payable to
Account Institution	**Account Institution**
Account #	Account #
Amount	Amount
Date of Transaction	Date of Transaction
For Deposit, Received from	For Deposit, Received from
For Withdrawal, Payable to	For Withdrawal, Payable to

Fig. 14.5 (continued)

Acknowledging and respecting wishes for burial, cremation, body and organ donation, gifts in memory of the deceased, and arrangements for memorial service and funerals are important considerations for the individual and family. Planning greatly reduces the difficulty of decisions through the guidance provided in documents drafted in advance of these critical life events.

An advance directive for healthcare informs family members, caregivers, and providers about patient preferences for care, which is particularly useful if the patient is unable or unwilling to make a healthcare decision (e.g., the patient is unconscious). Other advance care planning documents include (1) a living will, which indicates care preferences; (2) an appointment of healthcare agent, which

Documents	General Guidelines for How long to keep
Adoption Papers	For life
Bank Statements	6 years
Birth Certificates	For life
Business agreements	For life
Canceled checks	6 years
Contracts	Until updated
Credit Card Account Numbers	Until updated
Divorce papers	For life
Home purchase/improvement records	As long a s you own the property
Household inventory	Until updated
Insurance, life	For life
Insurance, Car, Home, etc.	Until updated
Investment Records	6 years after tax deadline for year of sale
Investment certificates	Until cashed or sold
Loan agreements	Unt il updated
Marriage certificate	For life
Military service records	For life
Mortgage papers	As long as you own the property
Real estate deeds	As long as you own the property
Receipts for large purchases	Until sale or discard
Service contracts/warranti es	Until sale or discard
Social Security card	For life
Tax returns	6 years from filing date
Vehicle titles	Until sale or disposal
Will	Until updated

Fig. 14.6 Important papers to keep and for how long

designates an agent or proxy; and (3) the portable directive or medical order, which provides documentation to healthcare providers and emergency medical service (EMS) personnel regarding the patient's wishes.

The following are explanations of the documents and associated terms commonly used for this type of planning. The appendix contains a link to resources for state-specific advance directive forms.

Advance Directives: Glossary of Terms

Cardiopulmonary resuscitation (CPR) — Steps taken when a person's heart stops. It can include compressions on the chest, electrical shocks, and breathing machines.

Do-not-resuscitate (DNR) order	Issued by a physician at the patient's request, a DNR orders EMS personnel and other providers not to try CPR if a person's heart or breathing stops.
Durable power of attorney for healthcare	A paper writing in which the patient appoints an agent who is authorized to make healthcare decisions for the patient. The document is also called a *healthcare proxy*.
Healthcare surrogate	Sometimes referred to as a *healthcare agent*. A surrogate is an individual, other than a patient's agent or guardian, who is authorized by state law to make a healthcare decision for the patient. The surrogate can make healthcare decisions for a patient if the patient is determined by a physician to lack capacity and no other healthcare agent or guardian has been appointed or is not reasonably available. If an individual lacks capacity and has not named an agent, or whose agent is not reasonably available, a surrogate will be identified by the supervising healthcare provider.

A surrogate must be an adult. The state statute will designate those persons to consider for surrogate in descending order of preference, such as the patient's spouse unless legally separated, adult child, parent, adult sibling, any other adult relative, or any other adult who has special care and concern for the patient or is familiar with the patient's personal values and is available and willing to serve.

Criteria for determining surrogate:

(a) Proposed surrogate reasonably appears to be better able to make decisions in accordance with the wishes of the patient or in accordance with the best interest of the patient.
(b) Proposed surrogate's regular contact with the patient prior to and during incapacitating illness.
(c) Proposed surrogate's availability to visit the patient during the illness.
(d) Proposed surrogate's availability to engage in face-to-face contact with healthcare providers to participate fully in the decision-making process.

If there are no eligible surrogates available, the designated physician may be authorized to make healthcare decisions for the patient after consultation with and recommendations of an institution's ethics board/committee/mechanism. The designated physician may be required to obtain concurrence from a second physician not directly involved in the patient's healthcare or not having close ties to the designated physician.

Depending upon state law, a decision to withhold or withdraw artificial nutrition and hydration can be made if the designated physician and a second independent physician certify in the patient's current clinical record that the provision or continuation of artificial nutrition/hydration is prolonging the act of dying, and if the patient is unlikely to regain capacity to make medical decisions, the surrogate may then make this healthcare decision on behalf of the patient.

Home care	Health services that are provided in the patient's home. These can be both skilled and non-skilled services, as defined by Medicare and other insurance benefits.
Hospice care	Hospice care is focused on relieving pain and emotional and spiritual support. It is provided to patients who are terminally ill and elect to forego therapeutic or curative care. Hospice care may be provided at home or in a residential or care facility. Hospice is a Medicare Part A benefit.
Intubation	Inserting a tube down a person's throat to help with breathing.
Palliative care	Palliative care is focused on relieving pain and stress. It may be administered in conjunction with therapeutic or curative care. Palliative care can be provided in hospitals, nursing homes, outpatient palliative care clinics, and certain other specialized clinics or at home. Medicare, Medicaid, and insurance policies may cover palliative care.
Percutaneous endoscopic gastrostomy (PEG) tube	Inserting a tube into the stomach to provide food and water.
Resuscitation	Steps taken when a person's heart stops. It can include compressions on the chest, electrical shocks, and breathing machines.
Ventilator	A machine that breathes for a patient who is otherwise unable to breathe.

POST (Physician's Orders for Scope of Treatment) Form

Available in most states, the POST form is a standardized form containing orders by a physician who has personally examined a patient regarding that patient's preferences for end-of-life care to address resuscitation and other end-of-life care services. In some states, this is called a POLST (Physician's Orders for Life-Sustaining Treatment) or MOLST (Medical Orders for Life-Sustaining Treatment) form. Figure 14.7 provides an example of a POST form.

Directions for Health Care Professionals

Completing POST

Must be completed by a health care professional based on patient preferences, patient best interest, and medical indications.

To be valid. POST must be signed by a physician or, at discharge or transfer from a hospital or long term care facility, by a nurse practitioner (NP), clinical nurse specialist (CNS), or physician assistant (PA). Verbal orders are acceptable with follow-up signature by physician in accordance with facility/community policy.

Person with DNR in effect at time of discharge must have POST completed by health care facility prior to discharge and copy of POST provided to qualified medical emergency personnel.

Photocopies/faxes of signed POST forms are legal and valid.

Using POST

Any incomplete section of POST implies full treatment for that section.

No defibrillator (including AEDs) should be used on a person who has chosen "Do Not Attempt Resuscitation".

Oral fluids and nutrition must always be offered if medically feasible.

When comfort cannot be achieved in the current setting, the person, including someone with "Comfort Measures Only", should be transferred to a setting able to provide comfort (e.g., treatment of a hip fracture).

IV medication to enhance comfort may be appropriate for a person who has chosen "Comfort Measures Only".

Treatment of dehydration is a measure which prolongs life. A person who desires IV fluids should indicate "Limited Interventions" or "Full Treatment".

A person with capacity, or the Health Care Agent or Surrogate of a person without capacity, can request alternative treatment.

Reviewing POST

This POST should be reviewed if:

(1) The patient is transferred from one care setting or care level to another, or
(2) There is a substantial change in the patient's health status, or
(3) The patient's treatment preferences change.

Draw line through sections A through D and write "VOID" in large letters if POST is replaced or becomes invalid.

COPY OF FORM SHALL ACCOMPANY PATIENT WHEN TRANSFERRED OR DISCHARGED.

Fig. 14.7 Physician's Order for Scope of Treatment (POST)

A COPY OF THIS FORM SHALL ACCOMPANY PATIENT WHEN TRANSFERRED OR DISCHARGED	
Tennessee Physician Orders for Scope of Treatment (POST, sometime called "POLST")	Patient's Last Name
This is a Physician Order Sheet based on the medical conditions and wishes of the person identified at right ("patient"). Any section not completed indicates full treatment for that section. When need occurs, first follow these orders, then contact physician.	First Name/Middle Initial
	Date of Birth

Section A *Check One Box Only*	**CARDIOPULMONARY RESUSCITATION (CPR): Patient has no pulse and is not breathing.** ☐ **Resuscitate (CPR)** ☐ **Do Not Attempt Resuscitation (DNR / no CPR) (Allow Natural Death)** When not in cardiopulmonary arrest, follow orders in **B**, **C**, and **D**.
Section B *Check One Box Only*	**MEDICAL INTERVENTIONS. Patient has pulse and/or is breathing.** ☐ **Comfort Measures Only.** Relieve pain and suffering through the use of any medication by any route, positioning, wound care and other measures. Use oxygen, suction and manual treatment of airway obstruction as needed for comfort. **Do not transfer to hospital for life-sustaining treatment. Transfer only if comfort needs cannot be met in current location. Treatment Plan: Maximize comfort through symptom management.** ☐ **Limited Additional Interventions.** In addition to care described in Comfort Measures Only above, use medical treatment, antibiotics, IV fluids and cardiac monitoring as indicated. No intubation, advanced airway interventions, or mechanical ventilation. May consider less invasive airway support (e.g. CPAP, BiPAP). **Transfer** to hospital if indicated. Generally avoid the intensive care unit. **Treatment Plan: basic medical treatment.** ☐ **Full Treatment.** In addition to care described in Comfort Measures Only and Limited Additional Interventions above, use intubation, advanced airway interventions, and mechanical ventilation as indicated. **Transfer** to hospital and/or intensive care unit if indicated. **Treatment Plan: Full treatment including in the intensive care unit.** *Other Instructions:*______
Section C *Check One*	**ARTIFICIALLY ADMINISTERED NUTRITION. Oral fluids & nutrition must be offered if feasible.** ☐ No artificial nutrition by tube. ☐ Defined trial period of artificial nutrition by tube. ☐ Long-term artificial nutrition by tube. *Other Instructions:*______

Section D *Must be Completed*	**Discussed with:** ☐ Patient/Resident ☐ Health care agent ☐ Court-appointed guardian ☐ Health care surrogate ☐ Parent of minor ☐ Other: ______(Specify)	**The Basis for These Orders Is:** (Must be completed) ☐ Patient's preferences ☐ Patient's best interest (patient lacks capacity or preferences unknown) ☐ Medical indications ☐ (Other) ______

Physician/NP/CNS/PA Name (Print)	Physician/NP/CNS/PA Signature Date NP/CNS/PA (Signature at Discharge)	MD/NP/CNS/PA Phone Number: ( )

Signature of Patient, Parent of Minor, or Guardian/Health Care Representative

Preferences have been expressed to a physician and /or health care professional. It can be reviewed and updated at any time if your preferences change. If you are unable to make your own health care decisions, the orders should reflect your preferences as best understood by your agent/surrogate.

Name (Print)	Signature	Relationship (write "self" if patient)	
Agent/Surrogate	Relationship	Phone Number ( )	
Health Care Professional Preparing Form	Preparer Title	Phone Number ( )	Date Prepared

Fig. 14.7 (continued)

Ethical Will

A document that is used to share the individual's values, beliefs, and blessings with family and community. It is not a legal document.

Living Will

A paper document that indicates care preferences if the individual is terminally ill or in a persistent vegetative state and there is no reasonable expectation of recovery. Signing with the statutory formalities typically required for a will, the individual may direct that his or her life not be artificially prolonged by artificial or extraordinary measures. A living will is the most inflexible of advance directives, as it attempts to set out detailed instructions pertaining to future unknown conditions with unknown medical treatments. Numerous living will forms are available, some that reflect particular value statements (such as Catholicism or Judaism).

Last Will and Testament

Most wills are similar in their basic contents. What often differs are the details pertaining to disposition of assets. What follows is a simple explanation of the basic parts of a will.

The first part of a will states who the maker of the will is. This individual is often referred to as the "testator." (A person who dies without a will dies "intestate.") The testator will name family members – spouse and children – and, if the testator has minor children, the testator will name the guardian of the children.

The next part of the will names the testator's "personal representative/executor." This is the person whom the testator entrusts to wind up his/her affairs and distribute the estate to the individual's beneficiaries. Here, the testator directs this personal representative to pay the testator's debts, including funeral expenses, as soon as possible.

The next part of the will is the "heart" of the will. This is where the testator makes bequests of his/her property. Most wills provide that beneficiaries divide personal property (called "tangible personal property").

If the will includes provisions for establishing a trust, those provisions will be written down at this part of the will. The testator will have named a trustee to hold the property in trust for the testator's beneficiaries (such as a spouse or a child with special needs). The paragraphs that would thereafter follow discuss the powers granted to the testator's trustee to hold and manage the trust property and the limitations on the trust.

The trust must also name the beneficiaries, how distributions are made and in what proportions, and how the trust terminates. If the will includes a trust, all of these requirements will be included.

Lastly, the will states how all other property in the testator's estate will be distributed. This is called the "residuary clause" and is included to make sure that if there is anything left in the estate, someone gets it.

One important provision in the will that the individual should be aware of appears here. This is the "written memorandum" paragraph. This paragraph authorizes the individual to make special bequests of personal property by a document separate from the will. To be a legal document, the written memorandum must be written out entirely in the testator's own handwriting, signed by the testator, and dated.

At the end of the will is place for the testator's signature. The two persons who witnessed the will have signed affidavits as well. This means that they will not have to appear in probate court to prove that this is the testator's will. Without these affidavits, it is possible that the court would be unable by law to admit the will to probate.

Probate: Briefly Explained

The purpose of writing a will is to make sure that the individual's intentions are carried out as set out in the will. The probate court's job is to ensure that the decedent's personal representative carries out the decedent's wishes.

Upon the individual's death, the decedent's personal representative will present the will to the probate court and receive the authority to handle the decedent's affairs and administer the decedent's estate.

Administration is largely an accounting job. The personal representative accounts for what is in the estate at the time of death, pays the lawful claims against the estate, and pays out the balance as the decedent's will directs or as the law provides. The personal representative can enter bank boxes and accounts, sell cars and trucks, transfer or sell stocks and bonds, and collect insurance proceeds payable to the estate.

When the personal representative has satisfactorily completed these tasks, the personal representative must go back to the probate court and make a final accounting of his or her duties. This final accounting will end the personal representative's job as administrator.

In most states, administration of an estate usually takes no more than 12 months. This does not mean that the beneficiaries cannot receive any of their inheritance before the estate is closed. This length of time is necessary to allow the decedent's creditors a period of time prescribed by the state's probate statute to file claims against the decedent's estate. For example, some states require creditors to file their claims within 6 months of the date that a notice to creditors is run a local newspaper. If all of the creditors are known and bills paid, the personal representative can make distributions of the estate to the designated beneficiaries.

Attorney-in-Fact (AIF)

An individual designated in instrument to act as agent of the principal granting powers of attorney.

Power of Attorney (POA)

An instrument/document granting someone authority to act as agent or attorney-in-fact for the grantor.

Durable Power of Attorney (DPOA)

A power of attorney that remains in effect notwithstanding the grantor's incompetency or incapacity.

Guardian/Conservator

The person who has been appointed by a judge to take care of a minor child or incompetent adult (both called a "ward") personal affairs and/or manage that person's financial affairs is called a "guardian" or "conservator." To become a guardian of a child, either the party intending to be the guardian or another family member, a close friend, or a local official responsible for a minor's welfare will petition the court to appoint the guardian. In the case of a minor, the guardianship remains under court supervision until the child reaches the age of majority.

Naming someone in a will as guardian of one's child in case of the death of the parent is merely a nomination. The judge does not have to honor that request, although he/she usually does. Sadly, often a parent must petition to become the guardian of his/her child's "estate" if the child inherits or receives a gift of substantial assets, including the situation in which a parent gives his/her own child an interest in real property or stocks. Therefore, that type of gift should be avoided and a trust created instead.

In some states, the term "guardian" applies to minors; and the term "conservator" applies to adults. While the term "guardian" may refer to someone who is appointed to care for and/or handle the affairs of a person who is incompetent or incapable of administering his/her affairs, this person may be called a "conservator" under a conservatorship.

Capacity

Capacity refers to an individual's ability to understand the significant benefits, risks, and alternatives, to proposed healthcare, and to make and communicate a decision. Assessment of decision-making capacity is critical in determining who will be making treatment decisions. Patients with decision-making capacity should make decisions for themselves; but if not, healthcare providers will need to rely on a surrogate decision-maker such as a healthcare agent. Decision-making capacity is the ability to understand and appreciate the consequences of health decisions and communicate a decision concerning healthcare in a meaningful manner.

Cognitive ability is related to capacity but is not the same thing. There is no definitive test for capacity. Capacity or the lack thereof can vary. Patients can have deficits in orientation, memory, recall, or attention span and still have capacity to make decisions. Capacity should also be thought of as existing on a continuum. Patients may have capacity to make some decisions but not others.

Although both describe ability to make decisions, decision-making capacity and legal competence are not the same thing. Capacity is a clinical determination. The evaluation involved in determining financial decision-making capacity is discussed in Chap. 6.

Competence/Incompetence

Competency is a legal determination. Patients are presumed competent until adjudicated incompetent.

Undue Influence

The improper use of power or trust in a way that deprives a person of free will and substitutes another's objective.

Privacy

Personal medical information is protected under the Health Insurance Portability and Accountability Act (HIPAA). The individual's permission is required to permit sharing of health information with family members.

HIPAA Standards

The *Standards for Privacy of Individually Identifiable Health Information* ("Privacy Rule") establishes a set of national standards for the protection of certain health information, known as the Health Insurance Portability and Accountability Act ("HIPAA").

Protected health information (includes individually identifiable health information) is information (including demographic data) that relates to:

- The individual's past, present, or future physical or mental health or condition
- The provision of healthcare to the individual
- The past, present, or future payment for the provision of healthcare to the individual

Table: Protected health information and HIPAA – circumstances where HIPAA may or may not apply

Situation	HIPAA protected Consent required	HIPAA not applicable
Routine medical treatment	X	
Mental health treatment	X	
Emergency medical treatment		X
Medical research participation	X	
Required by law: public health, law enforcement		X

Disclaimer

An advance directive is not a substitute for medical, legal, or other necessary advice or direction. These documents should not be construed as offering counseling; medical, legal, financial, or estate planning or advice; nor any other similar guidance or direction. Such counsel should be obtained from qualified, certified, and licensed professionals in your locale who are experienced in the specific areas of concern. Completion of these documents constitutes acceptance of its content both in whole and in part, as well as a determination of its utility for the purposes indicated.

Springer publisher and all involved in this document's design, publication, and distribution assume no liability for its use, including that which may arise from omissions, technical inaccuracies, and typographical errors.

Diligent efforts notwithstanding, this document is not warrantied to be in compliance with state and local laws. All warranties, including those of merchantability, fitness for a particular purpose, and non-infringement, are expressly disclaimed. The reader/user agrees to seek appropriate outside counsel prior to completion. The reader/user and all heirs, assigns, designees, devisees, representatives, and all others involved agree to assume all liability for its use and any subsequent outcomes and to release and hold harmless all involved in its design, publication, advertising, and distribution. The reader/user also agrees that any physician, healthcare provider, agent, proxy, surrogate, representative, mediator, court officer, and all others relying on the document's content are similarly free of all liability, when they act in good faith and with due diligence to follow the recorded wishes and directions.

References

1. U. S. Social Security Administration. What's Medicare? https://www.medicare.gov/what-medicare-covers/your-medicare-coverage-choices/whats-medicare. Accessed 4 Sept 2019.
2. U. S. Department of Health and Human Services. Medicaid. https://www.medicaid.gov/medicaid/index.html. Accessed 4 Sept 2019.
3. Centers for Medicare and Medicaid Services. What's Medicare supplement (Medigap) insurance? https://www.medicare.gov/supplements-other-insurance/whats-medicare-supplement-insurance-medigap. Accessed 4 Sept 2019.
4. Smith KB, Greenblatt A, Buntin J. Governing states and localities. Washington: A division of Congressional Quarterly, Inc.; 2005. p. 485.
5. Smith KB, Greenblatt A, Buntin J. Governing states and localities. Washington: A division of Congressional Quarterly, Inc.; 2005. p. 487.

Resources

A list of resources is provided for further background information and as examples for personalizing forms and directives.

AARP. Advance Directives Forms. https://www.aarp.org/caregiving/financial-legal/free-printable-advance-directives/. Accessed 4 Sept 2019.

Find state-specific advance directive forms which can be freely downloaded and completed.

American Bar Association. Pocket guide on elder investment fraud and financial exploitation. https://www.americanbar.org/content/dam/aba/publications/bifocal/BIFOCALNov-Dec2015.pdf. Accessed 4 Sept 2019.

Legal information to prevent financial fraud and abuse.

Centers for Medicare and Medicaid Services, Department of Health and Human Services. Medicare and you handbook. www.medicare.gov/Publications/Pubs/pdf/10050.pdf. Accessed 4 Sept 2019.

This informative handbook is written and distributed annually to all Medicare beneficiaries. It contains information on all the Medicare programs, which includes Parts A, B, C, and D.

Council on Aging of Greater Nashville, 2018 https://www.coamidtn.org/. Accessed 4 Sept 2019. Find helpful information on aging and caregiving, preventing scams, and a directory of community resources for seniors. Other communities may have councils on aging with similar guides adapted to local resources.

Department of Veterans Affairs Geriatrics and Extended Care website. https://www.va.gov/geriatrics/. Accessed 4 Sept 2019.

Excellent resource for veterans and their families regarding benefits, resources, and caregiver assistance. Provides links to many additional resources.

Five Wishes. Aging with dignity 2019. https://agingwithdignity.org/. Accessed 4 Sept 2019.

Easy-to-use legal advance directive document written in everyday language.

Morris V, Hansen JC. How to care for aging parents. NY: Workman Publishers; 2014.

A one-stop resource for medical, financial, housing, and emotional Issues.

Chapter 15
Methods to Protect Individuals from Financial Exploitation

Ronan M. Factora

Introduction

Older persons are very attractive targets for financial exploitation. There are a number of reasons for this. In the United States, persons over the age of 50 control over 70% of the nation's wealth. Seniors often undervalue their assets (e.g., they are often unaware that their homes have appreciated markedly). They often live with predictable daily patterns. For example, because these individuals likely receive monthly checks, abusers can predict when that person will have money on hand or need to go to the bank. People in this age group are dependent on others for assistance in many of their activities of daily living as a result of disabilities, allowing access for helpers to their homes and assets. Those with severe impairment are less likely to take action against their abusers as a result of illness or embarrassment. Some of them are unsophisticated about financial matters. Not surprisingly, advances in technology have made managing finances more complicated for older persons.

Caregivers may exercise significant influence over their victims. Abusers often assume frail victims will not survive long enough to follow through on legal interventions or that they will not make convincing witnesses.

For persons at risk of financial exploitation, preventing these events from happening is paramount in preserving their assets, independence, and financial stability in the community.

R. M. Factora (✉)
Cleveland Clinic Lerner College of Medicine at Case Western Reserve University, Cleveland Clinic, Cleveland, OH, USA
e-mail: factorr@ccf.org

R. M. Factora (ed.), *Aging and Money*,
https://doi.org/10.1007/978-3-030-67565-3_15

Who Is at Risk?

Determining who is at risk is a key step in preventing exploitation. Once risk is identified, steps can be taken to help prevent financial exploitation, identify clues that may suggest that financial exploitation is taking place, activate surveillance mechanisms to identify potential sources of exploitation, or initiate investigations when exploitation is thought to be taking place.

Several chapters in this book go into these topics in detail. Please refer to the following chapters for associated information:

- Chap. 3: Barriers to Recognition of Financial Exploitation
- Chap. 4: Risk Factors: The Individual and the Caregiver
- Chap. 5: Aging and Financial Risk

Victims of financial exploitation share many common characteristics. These individuals are often of older age, often women, and many are living alone. They are often trustful of others (even strangers), may be financially insecure (may require additional income) and lonely, and have a sense of trust/charity (a virtue that con artists will often take advantage of).

At-risk individuals may often not recognize that they are being exploited. It then falls on individuals who spend time with them to recognize that this is taking place.

Who Are the Perpetrators?

Perpetrators of abuse can be any individual, ranging from family members to close friends, acquaintances, or complete strangers. They can be professionals (who have a critical role in an individual's life) or the caregiver who comes in to take care of this person only a few hours weekly. Most often though, the perpetrators are family members.

Perpetrators often also share many common characteristics:

- A personal history of substance abuse, gambling, or financial problems.
- Fear of being deprived of an inheritance should the reported victim uses up savings.
- A history of untreated mental health issues.
- A sense of entitlement: These individuals are often used to living off of the reported victim. They may also stand to inherit from this individual and may feel justified in taking what they believe is "almost" or "rightfully" theirs. They may wish to prevent other family members from acquiring or inheriting from this individual as well.
- Opportunity: The relationship between the perpetrator and the victim may begin by honestly helping and then develops into appropriating the resources as their own.

Predatory strangers may actively seek out vulnerable seniors with the intent of exploiting them. Their goal is to obtain access into the home for the opportunity to access assets and property. Some of their actions to achieve this goal may include:

- Professing to love the reported victim ("sweetheart scams")
- Seeking employment by the individual (e.g. personal care attendants, counselors/advisers)
- Finding individuals who are recently widowed persons through newspaper death announcements or frequenting banks, malls, and restaurants to strike up friendships
- Advertising or answering ads on the Internet to be roommates

These individuals may move from community to community to avoid being apprehended.

Unscrupulous professionals or businesspersons or persons posing as such may take advantage of vulnerable elders by:

- Overcharging for services or products
- Using deceptive or unfair business practices
- Using their positions of trust or respect to gain compliance

Scams and forms of fraud perpetrated by such individuals are varied and creative. The following section details the most commonly encountered examples.

Examples of Types of Fraud

Older persons are common victims of individuals seeking to obtain access to their personal information, monies, and property. Perpetrators conduct these schemes using various recognized methods. Many local, state, and national government agencies have published brochures and information in paper and online to educate the general public about the types of fraud commonly used on the elderly. Often, this information is accompanied by ways that individuals can protect themselves from these forms of victimization.

The ultimate goal of these unscrupulous individuals is to acquire assets. Aside from cash and jewelry, this may also include life insurance benefits, pensions, annuities, "nest eggs," home equity, and property. In these schemes, the victim often cooperates with the perpetrator.

Fraud may go unrecognized for some time until the victim, family members, or friends recognize indicators that it is taking place. Clues that individual is being financially exploited include the following:

Loss of resources and assets:

- Insufficient funds to provide care for the older adult or level of care not commensurate with the individual's estate

- Loans taken out for necessary items
- Unpaid bills, utilities; associated notices for eviction or discontinuation of utilities
- Sudden changes in documents such as wills, powers of attorney, and other financial documents
- Disappearing items, including valuables, money (including unexplained transfers from bank accounts), credit cards, and assets

Changes in habits in managing financial affairs:

- A change in banking or spending habits, including excessive use of ATM or credit cards (particularly for non-care-related items)
- An increase in the number of checks made out to "cash"
- Irregularities noted on tax returns
- Financial statements and cancelled checks no longer coming to the older person's home
- A caregiver's name added to bank accounts and credit cards
- Discovery of an older individual's forged signature on checks, financial transaction documents, documents/titles related to possessions
- Individual is not allowed to spend money on what he/she wants or needs

Changes in behavior of the victim:

- A lack of knowledge/documentation or anxiety about financial status, financial transactions, status of documents (as above), location of monies or valuables
- The appearance of "new best friends"
- Reports assuming financial responsibility for adult family or friends
- Demonstration of fear, intimidation/threats, or submissiveness to a caregiver or another person
- Changes in behavior (isolated, withdrawn, depressed) or appearance (weight loss, poor hygiene) of the individual that is uncharacteristic
- Decline in the ability to perform activities of daily living independently
- Sudden change in residence
- Asks for "permission" from somebody to make a purchase or spend money
- Isolation from family, friends, community, or other stable relationships
- Missed appointments
- Home filled with sweepstake, junk mail, magazines, and unopened "gifts"

Changes in behavior of the caregiver:

- Frequent/expensive gifts from individual to caregiver.
- Caregiver is noted to be spending excessive amounts of money on jewelry and personal items.
- Caregiver will not allow the individual to be alone with a physician or other family members.

- Excessive interest in financial status paid by caregiver or other individuals.
- Implausible explanations given about the elderly person's finances by the elder or the caregiver.
- Misuse of power of attorney or guardianship by not acting in the best interests of the individual for whom this resposibility was granted.

Perpetrators of financial exploitation can be creative in developing a means of obtaining an older person's assets. These methods can be divided into several categories:

- Scams: Typically these are scenarios where items or services are given in exchange for money, property, or other assets. Often these items and services are unrealistic and fake, or the cost exceeds the true value of the service or item. Table 15.1 describes some commonly encountered scams.

Table 15.1 Commonly encountered scams and how to avoid them

Credit repair scams: These scams are sold as a means to improve personal credit by erasing bad credit, lowering interest rates, and consolidating debts. Often, individuals are charged hundreds or thousands of dollars for these services that do not provide the benefit promised
How to avoid: Contact a nonprofit credit counseling agency or creditors directly to get help. This is often a free service.
Fake check scams: In this scenario, an individual is sent a check or money order which the mailer asks to be deposited, with a portion of the money wire-transferred to the sender. The incentive to the individual is that a portion of this money is supposed to remain in their personal account. In reality, the check or money order is usually counterfeit, and it will be returned to your bank unpaid, with a full amount deducted from your account
How to avoid: Never wire-transfer money to a stranger
Advance fee loans: Individuals are told that they qualify for a loan or credit card after paying a "fee." Scammers offer a line of credit or state that the money will be direct deposited into the bank account once this fee is paid. In the end, there typically is no loan, credit card, or any money
How to avoid: Do not pay advance fees for a credit card or a loan
Prizes/sweepstakes/foreign lottery scams: Individuals are told they have won the lottery, a contest of some sort but often are asked to pay a fee to collect their winnings. Victims will send money via wire transfer or money order (sometimes to a foreign country). Despite being told when to expect their winnings, the prize never arrives
How to avoid: Legitimate sweepstakes are free and do not require wire transfers. Once again, paying advance fees is never recommended. Keep credit card and bank account numbers safe and private – avoid sharing. This information may be requested during an unsolicited sales pitch and could be used to access and empty bank accounts
Family and caregiver rescue scams: Perpetrators in this type of scam are typically family members, caregivers, or friends. In asking for financial assistance, these individuals may use the older person's credit card, have them sign over a power of attorney for finances, or forge their signatures on checks or other financial documents
How to avoid: Prevention can be difficult, but there are signs that a scam is taking place that should be watched for. These may include a senior's bills going unpaid, getting a new "best friend," that older person being excluded or cut off to access from other family members or friends, showing a pattern of unusual banking activities, or missing belongings

(continued)

Table 15.1 (continued)

Grandparent scams: This scam takes advantage of close relationships between grandparents and their grandchildren. Con artists posing as grandchildren make a story saying they are in trouble, sometimes stuck in another country, and require money that needs to be immediately wired to them. The grandparent will send the money to location provided, but the money will instead go to the con artists and not to the intended/impersonated grandchild
How to avoid: Callers should always be asked to be identified by name. Asking the caller a question that only family members would know the answer to will help determine if the caller is who they say they are. Personal information should not be volunteered over the phone. Calling the friend or relative claiming to need your help can confirm whether the story is true, particularly when calling that person using a phone number known to be genuine. If contact with that person cannot be made, then an attempt should be made to call other friends or family members to confirm the situation. Requests for sending money via wire transfer should be refused. If money has been wired but has not been picked up yet, it is recommended to immediately call the wire transfer service and cancel the transaction. Once the money has been picked up, there is no way to get it back
Charity scams: In this scheme, scammers take advantage of the altruistic feelings of seniors. Mail and phone calls are used to obtain donations for various causes including helping out disabled veterans or friends in foreign countries, animal causes, or lobby Congress for senior benefits such as Social Security. The use of recent news events, providing the details about specific cases, and appealing emotionally to the victim are common ploys used by con artists. It can be difficult to determine how much of this money actually goes to the "cause" as many charities keep a large fraction of donations
How to avoid: Legitimacy of the charity should be verified before making any donation. Finding out how much of the money actually goes to the charitable purpose and how much goes to the cost of fundraising (you can ask the charity this directly when they call) gives a sense of how the money that is being donated is being spent
Foreclosure rescue scams: Homeowners having difficulty making her house payments are targets of this particular type of scam. These scammers typically make promises (as a phony foreclosure rescue company) to contact and negotiate with individual's lender to avoid foreclosure. The cost is often thousands of dollars, but this company makes little or no contact with a lender. In another scenario, an "investor" offers to purchase an individual's home and lease back until the mortgage payments can be made. In this situation, this "investor" takes the money, but there is no transfer of the mortgage loan nor is there payment to the lender. Consequently, the homeowner risks losing equity as well as ownership of the home
How to avoid: Foreclosure assistance is often available through reliable government agencies
Home improvement fraud: This often involves door-to-door contractors offering to repair, upgrade, or service a home. Many scam artists may also offer model home discounts, free inspections, or leftover supplies from repairs made to another home in the neighborhood. They may ask for a large down payment or money upfront, but often these contractors or companies do not complete work that they were paid to do or do a poor job
How to avoid: Large down payments should be avoided, and payment using cash or check should also be avoided – credit cards often offer protection if something goes wrong with the contract work. Calling the Better Business Bureau to research the contractor can help uncover any problems with them encountered by other individuals/parties. If planning to hire a contractor, it should be confirmed that the contractor is registered and bonded. The contractor's references should be checked, and several potential bids for the work requested should be solicited to get a full sense of how much the job should really cost (and avoid being overcharged by a single contractor)

Table 15.1 (continued)

Living trust scams: These are high-pressure sales, often targeting lower-income consumers, with a promise of avoiding probate costs or promoting the tax advantages of living trusts (these are legal arrangements for transferring assets into a trust while the consumer is still alive in order to keep such assets from going through probate court when the consumer dies). These claims from the scammer are often exaggerated; consumers are often unaware of other options for estate planning
How to avoid: Contacting an estate attorney or elder care attorney is recommended instead when choosing to arrange for a trust. These arrangements should not be made through door-to-door salespersons or telemarketers. The name and phone number of such professionals can be obtained by calling your local bar association or another lawyer referral service
Work-at-home/business opportunity ploys: In this scheme, individuals are asked to pay in advance for materials and startup costs to start businesses at home or to invest in a business opportunity. The scammers are often the only ones who profit and may utilize high-pressure sales pitches on their anticipated victims
How to avoid: Suspicion should be raised with companies promising regular market or steady income through this line of work. Paying for information about work-at-home offers (advance payment should not be a requirement for work to be done at home) is not recommended. Instead, the Better Business Bureau, the local Chamber of Commerce, or the State Attorney General's Office should be contacted prior to making any decisions about such offers. The details regarding this "opportunity" should be discussed with one of these organizations to ensure their legitimacy

- Identity theft: Use of name, personal identification information (Social Security number, date of birth, etc.), or account numbers (bank accounts, credit cards) to directly obtain money or to obtain loans and other lines of credit (based on in individual's good credit), receive medical treatment, get personal/private information/identification, or otherwise pretend to be the victim. Thieves, using the victim's name, could open new account, purchase products, and then leave the consumer to pay the bill. Phishing is the use of calls or e-mails to obtain such personal information. Perpetrators, often pretending to be a bank or government agency, ask to update or confirm account information by having the individual submit bank account numbers, passwords, or Social Security number.
- Insurance fraud: Individuals selling fake insurance policies.
- Reverse mortgage: This refers to the use of the equity in a home while still residing in it to obtain loans or for other personal needs. Though it is not a scam, high-pressure sales tactics could be used to take out reverse mortgages (which may be accompanied by very high fees). Sometimes other salespeople may encourage the use of this loan money to buy annuities or investments that may not provide any benefit.
- Predatory lending: The practice of encouraging individuals to take out unnecessary loans, often with no clear purpose, or to take advantage of an individual's financial situation (such as high interest rate loans for individuals to purchase a home or a car for another family member/friend/acquaintance).

There are some common characteristics to scams. If any of the following are seen, the targeted person could end up becoming a victim of fraud:

- The individual is asked to wire money to someone not known to them.
- The individual is notified that they are a winner of a contest that that person had never heard of or entered.
- The individual is placed under pressure to "act now!".
- A fee is required to receive a "prize".
- Personal information (social security number, PIN number, bank account information) is requested.
- The individual is asked to pay a large down payment.
- No written information is provided for the company that has contacted the individual.
- A company that has contacted the individual has no physical address – only a PO Box.

Action Plans

Though recognizing clues that exploitation may be taking place is important to prevent its success, taking protective steps is the best method of avoiding victimization. Often these interventions can be implemented before an event occurs. Knowing the resources available to assist the community to recognize and stop scams is also valuable.

Setting Up Protections from Financial Abuse

One recommendation is to make sure that individuals plan ahead. The more thought you put into future planning, then the greater control one has as a person gets older, even if that individual is no longer physically present of cognitive able to make these decisions:

- Consider prepaying for funeral arrangements and other services that may be needed someday.
- Document all financial arrangements.
- Put all of decisions in writing. This can help prevent future misunderstandings and legal problems.

Another recommendation is to hire the appropriate professionals to help with this planning. A Certified Public Accountant (CPA) or Certified Financial Planner (CFP) can help handle concerns including how much money can be safely withdrawn from retirement funds. Estate planning attorneys with elder law expertise can help write will and power of attorney documents and craft trusts (which can limit a potential beneficiary's access to money). A professional daily money manager can help deal with bill-paying, insurance claims, phone calls to financial institutions, and troubleshooting financial matters.

Consideration should be made to execute documents such as a will, living will, or durable healthcare power of attorney or financial power of attorney to appropriately plan for the future. Ideally, these documents should be drawn up while the individual is of sound mind and body and kept in a secure location (see Chap. 14 for more information regarding documents that should be considered as one gets older). They should clearly reflect that individual's wishes. A trusted adviser should be identified so that they also know where these documents are kept and how to access them if needed.

Power of attorney is a powerful position. Legally, this person is considered the fiduciary of the individual who has assigned them, and they charged with acting in the best interests of that individual. In practice, this individual could do anything with the money of the individual to which they have been assigned authority – assignment of this level of power should serve as a warning prior to giving any individual that legal designation. Sometimes the person considered "closest" to the individual concerned is not necessarily the best person to do the best job. It may be better assigning this responsibility to someone more detached and financially secure. Careful consideration should be given prior to assigning anyone this role.

With the above in mind, the power of attorney document can be drawn up with limits. This may include assigning a relative or friend to monitor the person designated as power of attorney, mandating a periodic written report of financial transactions. Joint powers of attorney may also be assigned, requiring two signatures on every check. Chores may be split, giving one person authority over financial matters and another control of health decisions. A lawyer of the persons concerned may be asked to hold the physical papers granting power of attorney, to help ensure that the appointee cannot prematurely present it to that person's investment company or bank to gain access at inappropriate or unnecessary times.

For persons considering making these assignments or completing these documents, it is a good idea to stay active within the community and with family. Developing a large network of friends and accumulating knowledge about places and organizations available to provide assistance can reduce the risk of abuse or exploitation. Maintaining good relationships with one's attorney, banker, and other professionals in the community can be useful in accessing important resources to help with planning and also having their perspectives available to be watchful for any signs of abuse or exploitation. Isolation can not only lead to loneliness and depression, but it also makes one more vulnerable to financial abuse or exploitation.

There are many ways to keep your assets secure and protected. The following methods are considered effective:

- Asking the bank for help in arranging who can access funds: Consideration should always made in deciding who is to be added to accounts, as that individual can access it at any time.

- Ensuring that signature cards and contact information are up to date and updated periodically.
- Continuously keeping track of finances by (1) reviewing bank statements carefully to make sure that all charges accurately reflect individual purchases and payments and (2) considering sending duplicate statements to a trusted advisor/family member who has no access to the accounts to watch for inaccuracies or fraud.
- Avoiding being pressured into withdrawing large amounts of money.
- Using direct deposit for all regular checks such as Social Security (this helps prevent mail theft).
- Arranging automated bill payments through the bank for mortgage payments, utility bills, and other regular expenses.
- Securing all blank checks to limit access.
- Avoiding signing the back of a check unless there is a plan to cash it immediately.
- Avoiding lending or displaying of identification cards, credit card, ATM cards, or checks to anyone.
- Cancelling ATM or credit cards that are unused.
- Getting free reports from the three major credit bureaus through www.annualcreditreport.com to check for unapproved loans, credit cards, etc.
- Using professionals (bank professionals, law enforcement, or social service agencies) to help handle money and review financial activities and identify concerning changes. It is always a good idea to ask for help from these professionals if an individual is being threatened, abused, or exploited.
- Being cautious about signing documents but specifically avoiding signing any documents that are not completely understood or which the individual is being pressured to sign.
- Avoiding sharing a large bank account or a credit card with another person. In circumstances where assistance is needed to help pay bills, a shared account could be arranged, BUT only enough money to pay the bills should be transferred to that account when appropriate.
- Getting to know officers and tellers at the local bank or credit union where an account is placed.
- Paying with a check, not cash, and always getting a receipt of the transaction.

Setting Up Protections for the Home

- Performing due diligence prior to hiring a contractor: Before finally hiring someone to do work in the home, it is recommended that that person's references be checked. It should not be assumed that a placement agency will do a thorough reference/background check. Instead, a national, rather than a state, criminal check should be conducted. Proof that the agency providing the hired individual is bonded should be requested, and this documentation should be confirmed with the local Better Business Bureau. To monitor in-home help, consider installing a surveillance camera if state law permits it. This seems like a lot of work, but it can help improve the chances of hiring a more reputable and responsible individual to do work around the home.

- Avoiding falling victim to phone scams and be assisted by subscribing to national and state Do-Not-Call lists.
- Setting up caller ID helps screen phone calls for telemarketers. The call record also allows other family members to see who has been calling the home and look for a pattern of phone calls.
- Shredding all financial documents and documents with identifying information prior to discarding can reduce the risk of private information falling into the hands of unscrupulous individuals.
- Avoiding leaving mail in an unsecured mailbox.
- Listing and photographing all jewelry and valuables, so they can be traced to pawn shops if necessary.
- Keeping small valuables in a locked drawer and photographs of them in a separate place.

It is important to guard personal information. Important information such as Social Security numbers, ATM cards, or PIN numbers should not be given to strangers or anyone who does not need them. Avoiding giving away this information over the phone is also important unless it is being given to a well-known and reputable company.

Caregiver/Family Interventions

Caregivers and family members can also act to protect vulnerable family members or others in the community from abuse. As caregivers may often develop strain and burnout, they should get breaks and obtain respite as burned-out caregivers are more likely to abuse care recipients. Recommending that a caregiver participates in a support group or seeks counseling through a licensed provider may be helpful when that person is feeling stressed or overwhelmed.

If there are paid caregivers or if a family member is in a facility, family members should remain involved and observant to make sure that the quality of care being delivered is appropriate and to watch for any signs of abuse or neglect. Though this happens very infrequently in aggregate living facilities, it is worthwhile to remain vigilant.

Family members can act proactively by providing tips to at-risk individuals regarding recently encountered telephone solicitations and other forms of fraud and scams that they may fall victim to. Advising family members to remain cautious when managing their finances and seeking assistance and counseling prior to making financial decisions may help avert situations where they may be taken advantage of. Providing knowledge about what is going on in the world and what resources are available to assist in making important financial decisions can only help protect a person from exploitation.

The most important action one can take on an older relative's behalf is to make sure he or she gets out and about. Elder abuse is correlated highly with social and physical isolation. In addition to family making regular and unplanned visits, arranging outings and visits with friends, neighbors, clergy, and volunteers helps prevent isolation. Socialization and participation in community gathering and activities help ensure that a number of people are watching each other and may be around to notice anything suspicious or concerning and act on it.

If there are concerns about how a family member is managing their financial affairs, it would be worthwhile to hold a family meeting to discuss who will look after that relative physically and financially. If one relative will handle the bulk of the care, it would be reasonable to have an attorney draft a "personal care agreement" that outlines how much he or she should receive for services. Laying out such ground rules can help avoid caregivers from taking advantage of individuals and also recognizes and acknowledges the amount of care being directed to the family member in need.

Setting up a limited account can be considered if there are concerns about a relative's ability to make financial decisions. This small account can be set up at a local bank and may include a debit card and checks that have a spending limit. Arrangements can be with the bank to investigate checks written for more than this limit. This arrangement can give that individual the freedom to access and spend their funds while preventing excessive losses.

Family members should be available to accompany their relatives to meetings with financial advisers and doctors. These professionals could be helpful in arranging and implementing plans to protect that family member's health and finances, and the presence of a trusted family member or caregiver can help ensure that the plan is implemented and followed through.

Caregivers or family suspecting abuse should discuss these concerns directly with the individual being victimized. That person should be encouraged to be open about their thoughts, feelings, and concerns now or at any time in the future. They should be reassured that family and friends are there to listen and assist in any possible way, support them through that difficult situation, and help maintain as much of their independence as possible.

Benefits of Preventative Interventions

Implementation of many of the previously stated interventions can be time-consuming and tedious, but they can prove to be extremely useful if an individual becomes a victim of some form of financial exploitation. Potentially, a paper trail can be followed that may demonstrate how transactions have been made contrary to the wishes of the individual being allegedly exploited, how long the exploitation has been taking place, what venues were sites of exploitation, and who the perpetrator may be. Evidence that may become useful in investigations includes the following items:

- Financial statements from a bank, credit card companies, or a brokerage firm
- Signature cards, account applications
- Checkbooks, check registers, deposit slips
- Personal photographs that show property or conditions before the reported perpetrator became involved
- Credit bureau information (to demonstrate the use of personal information to obtain loans or lines of credit)
- Legal documents (wills, powers of attorney, trusts)
- Documented change of mailing addresses, post office boxes
- Presence of catalogs and advertisements (may indicate shopping sprees)

Available Resources

Individuals should never feel that they are alone in protecting themselves or those they care for from financial abuse and exploitation. Identifying at-risk individuals and recognizing clues suggesting that abuse is occurring are already daunting tasks. A varied array of resources are available at local, regional, state, and national levels to help protect individuals from as well as act to investigate suspected financial exploitation. Table 15.2 lists a variety of these resources that should be accessed in these circumstances.

Scams should be reported to your State Attorney General's Office.

Table 15.2 Resources

Consumer Financial Protection Bureau's Office of Financial Protection for Older Americans: http://www.consumerfinance.gov/older-americans/ Receives and investigates consumer fraud complaints specifically related to mortgages, credit cards, banks, loans, and more
National Academy of Elder Law Attorneys: http://www.naela.org/ Offers a search for lawyers specializing in durable powers of attorney, conservatorship, estate planning, elder abuse, and other concerns
National Adult Protective Services Association (NAPSA): https://www.napsa-now.org/ Provides a national map with links to abuse-reporting hotlines by state
National Center on Elder Abuse (NCEA): https://ncea.acl.gov/ Has links to additional state directories of help lines, hotlines and elder-abuse prevention resources in all 50 states and the District of Columbia
National Committee for the Prevention of Elder Abuse (NCPEA): www.preventelderabuse.org provides information on all aspects of elder abuse. Its website has a designated section to help victims and those vulnerable to abuse, providing information in cases of suspected abuse, what services are available to stop it, and information about community resources. Search under "Elder Abuse," "Help for Victims and Vulnerable Persons"

(continued)

Table 15.2 (continued)

The National Association of Area Agencies on Aging (n4a): https://www.n4a.org/ The National Association of Area Agencies on Aging (n4a) is the umbrella organization for the 655 Area Agencies on Aging throughout the U.S. These Area Agencies on Aging provide information and services and coordinate and administer programs for older adults. The website provides contact information for your local Area Agency on Aging
AARP Money Management Program: https://www.aarp.org/aarp-foundation/our-work/income/ Pairs seniors of limited resources or people with disabilities with trained money-management volunteers. One service helps seniors who remain in control of their finances to balance their checkbooks and pay bills; the other focuses on those deemed incapable of handling their own funds. The program is offered in 21 states and the District of Columbia, though availability varies
American Association of Daily Money Managers: https://secure.aadmm.com/ Links seniors to members nationwide who can assist with bill-paying, banking, insurance paperwork, and organizing records in preparation for income-tax filing, among other tasks
National Association of Professional Geriatric Care Managers: https://www.aginglifecare.org/ Provides links to professionals who can facilitate aspects of seniors' lives, including monitoring home-care workers, managing medical appointments, and identifying potential exploitation risks, among other services. Additional services may include bill payment and handling medical/financial/legal paperwork
Better Business Bureau Scam Stopper: https://www.bbb.org/scamtips/ Has information on common scams and instructions on reporting a scam. Individuals can sign up for scam alerts
Investor Protection Trust: http: http://www.investorprotection.org/protect-yourself/?fa=protect-seniors An independent organization which provides information about elder fraud and methods of how to protect yourself from harm
National Do Not Call Registry: To register, call 1-888-382-1222 or going online to https://donotcall.gov/
Three major credit bureaus:
Equifax – https://www.equifax.com/personal/
To order your report, call: 800-685-1111 or write: P.O. Box 740241, Atlanta, GA 30374-0241
To report fraud, call: 800-525-6285 and write: P.O. Box 740241, Atlanta, GA 30374-0241
Hearing impaired call 1-800-255-0056 and ask the operator to call the Auto Disclosure Line at 1-800-685-1111 to request a copy of your report
Experian – https://www.experian.com/
To order your report, call: 888-EXPERIAN (397-3742) or write: P.O. Box 2002, Allen TX 75013
To report fraud, call: 888-EXPERIAN (397-3742) and write: P.O. Box 9530, Allen TX 75013
TTY: 1-800-972-0322
Trans Union – https://www.transunion.com/
To order your report, call: 800-888-4213 or write: P.O. Box 1000, Chester, PA 19022
To report fraud, call: 800-680-7289 and write: Fraud Victim Assistance Division, P.O. Box 6790, Fullerton, CA 92634
TTY: 1-877-553-7803
To request that they notify retailers who use their databases not to accept your checks, call:
TeleCheck: 1-800-710-9898 or 927-0188
Certegy, Inc. (previously Equifax Check Systems): 1-800-437-5120
To find out whether an identity thief has been passing checks in your name call: SCAN: 1-800-262-7771

Future Directions

Much of research conducted in the area of financial exploitation has explored its incidence, its prevalence, and who the victims are. As in most of the field of elder abuse, more studies need to be conducted to understand this issue in greater detail so as to identify risk factors for which preventative interventions may be effective. Several questions in this area need to be answered:

- What are the causes of financial exploitation?
- What are the measurable consequences for its victims?
- What characteristics of the victims put them at risk (including the presence of and severity of cognitive impairment) ?
- What characteristics of perpetrators make them more likely to conduct an act of financial exploitation?
- How can technology be leveraged to identify those at risk and protect them from exploitation?
- Is education of those at risk for exploitation helpful in reducing their risk?

Advancement of research in this field will aid those in the front lines who help the victims of financial exploitation to reach those at risk sooner and preserve the assets that these individuals rely upon to preserve their quality of life.

Index

© Springer Nature Switzerland AG 2021
R. M. Factora (ed.), *Aging and Money*,
https://doi.org/10.1007/978-3-030-67565-3